# COOLBEANS

**ONE WOMAN'S MISSION TO RECLAIM FERTILITY THROUGH MEN'S HEALTH**

# SAARA JAMIESON

Foreword Tory Trewhitt

Copyright © 2025
First Published in Australia in 2025
By Morpheus Publishing
Geelong Victoria 3216
www.morpheuspublishing.com.au

All rights reserved. No part of this publication may be reproduced, stored in a retrieval system, or transmitted in any form or by any means, electronic, mechanical, photocopying, recording or otherwise, without the prior written permission of the publisher or author.

Paperback ISBN: 978-1-7643352-0-1
Author: Saara Jamieson
Foreword: Tory Trewhitt
Cover Graphics: Mylen Carascal

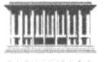

A catalogue record for this book is available from the National Library of Australia.

### DISCLAIMER
The information contained in this book is for general informational purposes only. The author and publisher are not offering any medical, legal or professional advice. While every effort has been made to ensure the accuracy and completeness of the information provided, the author and publisher assume no responsibility for errors or omissions or any outcomes or consequences resulting from using this book's content.

### COPYRIGHT
All original material in this book is the sole property of the author and Morpheus Publishing.

### DISTRIBUTION
This book is distributed by Morpheus Publishing and is available through authorised distributors, booksellers, Morpheus Publishing website.

### COPYRIGHT PERMISSIONS
For copyright permissions or any other inquiries, please contact:

**PUBLISHER: Morpheus Publishing**
www.morpheuspublishing.com.au  ||  hello@justinemartin.com.au  ||  +61403 564 942

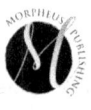

**AUTHOR: Saara Jamieson**
https://www.morpheuspublishing.com.au/authors/saara-jamieson

**DISCLAIMER:**

The information provided in this book is for general educational and informational purposes only. It is not intended as a substitute for professional medical advice, diagnosis, or treatment. Always seek the advice of your physician or other qualified healthcare provider with any questions you may have regarding a medical condition or health concerns.

While Cool Beans Underwear® is recommended based on research and personal experience, it should not be used as a sole solution for reproductive health or other men's health concerns. Cool Beans is a complementary product designed to assist with heat-related issues that may impact fertility and overall wellbeing. It is not intended to treat, cure, or prevent any medical condition. Individual results may vary, and what may have assisted one person may not assist others due to a variety of factors.

This book addresses a wide range of men's health issues, including fertility, hormone regulation, mental health, and longevity. While Cool Beans may support aspects of these, it should be considered part of a holistic approach to men's health. It is not a substitute for medical treatment or a comprehensive healthcare regimen.

Every effort has been made to provide accurate, up-to-date information. However, as new research becomes available, we cannot guarantee that the information in this book will remain current, and we take no responsibility for any incorrect or outdated material.

Please consult a healthcare professional before making any significant changes to your lifestyle, diet, or healthcare regimen. The author and publisher disclaim any liability for any adverse outcomes arising from following the advice or suggestions within this book.

# CONTENTS

How to use this book ................................................................ vii

This side of the story – Why I'm writing this book now ................ ix

Foreword .................................................................................... xi

Prologue: Where we are today .................................................... 1

Preface: The day I knew .............................................................. 9

**PART I: STARTING THE JOURNEY ........................................ 17**

Chapter 1: The wonder of what could be .................................... 19

Chapter 2: The day the line faded ............................................... 27

This side of the story – For our beloved Nanna Mitchell, and Aunty Kerry – our hearts are with you today and always. ..................... 35

Chapter 3: Six months of silence ................................................ 37

Chapter 4: This is routine ............................................................ 45

Chapter 5: Wine, fire and darkness ............................................. 53

This side of the story – Just finished writing part one of this book ... 59

Chapter 6: Jordan's story ........................................................... 61

**PART II: WHEN THE BALLS DROPPED ................................. 69**

Chapter 7: Mosquito netting and masculinity ............................... 71

# Contents

Chapter 8: Silent, curious, scared: The men who whisper .................. 79

Chapter 9: Boiling point ........................................................... 87

Chapter 10: Let's not f*ck this up .............................................. 95

This side of the story – This is bigger than underwear ..................... 102

## PART III: COOL BEANS AND THE NEW FRONTIER .................. 105

Chapter 11: The penis goes where?! The science behind the pouch that changed everything ........................................................... 107

Chapter 12: The canary in the coal mine..................................... 121

This side of the story – When the warning signs are right in front of us ........................................................................... 132

Chapter 13: The men we've met ................................................ 135

Chapter 14: What some women wish men knew ......................... 145

Chapter 15: What men wish they could say ................................. 153

This side of the story – Turning shame into power ........................ 162

## PART IV: THE SILENT EPIDEMIC .............................................. 165

Chapter 16: The cost of vision ................................................... 167

Chapter 17: Raising stronger sons ............................................. 179

This side of the story – Letter to my son: What strength really means ........................................................ 189

Chapter 18: And then came Heidi ............................................... 193

This side of the story – Letter to my daughter: My mission, your fire ............................................................... 204

Chapter 19: Sex, sperm & society .............................................. 207

## PART V: A NEW KIND OF STRENGTH ...................................... 221

Chapter 20: The future we're building ........................................ 223

This side of the story – The ripple effect .................................... 234

Chapter 21: Futureproofing manhood ................................................. 237

Chapter 22: Global blind spots ............................................................ 249

Chapter 23: For the children we're raising today or yet to come ...... 261

This side of the story – A world we are creating for our
children – and all of us .......................................................................... 275

Epilogue: The mission is just beginning ............................................. 279

Reader Reflection: What will you leave behind? ................................ 283

Bonus Section: Tools for change-makers ........................................... 291

References ............................................................................................. 297

# HOW TO USE THIS BOOK

This book is a mix of personal story, science, and straight talk – sometimes emotional, sometimes practical, always real.

While my story focuses on infertility, that's just one part of a much bigger picture: the accelerating decline of men's health. Testosterone, vitality, mental health, longevity – it's all connected, and it affects everyone. This isn't just about conception. It's about awareness, action, and hope. My journey is the starting point for a much-needed conversation.

Whether you're reading this because you've lived something similar, because you love someone who has, or because you simply want to understand what's happening – welcome. This book is for all of us. We all know and love men. We all care about the people closest to us – our partners, sons, brothers, fathers, and friends. Men's health isn't a niche issue. It shapes our families, our futures, and the world we're building for the next generation.

At the end of each chapter, you'll find a section called *Putting it into practice* – simple, actionable steps for you, your partner, or both of you together. These might seem small, but they're designed to help relationships weather tough times and support a healthier future – always grounded in science, never just opinion.

Following that is *Behind the chapter: Sources* – an optional section that lists the studies behind each chapter and, where useful, adds brief context to support the *Putting it into practice* items further. If you're here for the story, feel free to skip these; the chapter stands on its own. If you're curious, want the "why", or prefer to see the receipts, this section is for you.

You'll also see *This side of the story* – short, real-time reflections that appear throughout the book. Written in the moment or sparked by something in my present-day life, they offer a window into how this journey continues to unfold. Think of them as check-ins from the other side – a pause to reflect, reconnect, and breathe.

Please know I didn't get everything right. I am human – hopeful, sometimes wobbly, always learning. My hope is that this book gives you what I wish I'd had: a little more light, a little more clarity, and a little less loneliness.

If you're on a similar path – or even just curious – I hope this book makes your journey a little easier. And if it sparks one more conversation, one more action, one more shift – then it's already doing its job.

## THIS SIDE OF THE STORY
### – WHY I'M WRITING THIS BOOK NOW

Over the past six years, while slowly building Cool Beans Underwear®, the idea of writing a book has floated in and out of my mind more times than I can count. People would say, "You should write your story." And part of me always agreed.

But English was never my strong suit. Sure, there was one exception – in Grade 4, I wrote a short story called The Tree That Always Said No. It was about a grouchy old tree that refused every bird, animal, and child who wanted to make a home, forage food, or climb in its branches. Eventually, the world gave up on it. The tree grew tall, strong... and was all alone. The tree became lonely and sad. Until one day, a boy asked, "Can I hang my swing in your big, strong branch?" And for the first time, the tree said "yes". That story placed second in the district, and I won $100. I was nine years old and oh so proud.

But after that? I was a steady B-C student in English. English and writing were never things I felt particularly good at. Despite this, the dream of writing a book quietly stayed with me, tucked away behind deadlines, business plans, and the constant juggle of life.

For those who don't know, I was recently invited to contribute a chapter to Dreams and Determination, a collection of stories from inspirational women founders. Writing that chapter showed me that I was capable of creating something people wanted to read. More importantly, it gave me the space to reflect on how far I've come – how far Jordan and I have come – and how far we've come together as a family. And that maybe, just maybe, my voice and story do belong on the page.

Around that same time, I reached out to Andrew Jobling – former St Kilda AFL player (for non-Australian readers, that stands for Australian Football League) and host of The Wellness Puzzle podcast

– to ask if I could be a guest on his show ahead of Men's Health Week 2025. I'll never forget the look on his face when I asked. I think he thought I was about to pitch him to help write my book – which he does for many authors, and also now for me. But I didn't. I asked to share my story. Maybe he was surprised by how direct I was. Maybe he was proud that his platform had reached a place where people were coming to him. Either way, it sparked something that stayed with me.

Because after that conversation, something shifted. Andrew didn't just hear my story – he saw it. He saw why it mattered. And in doing so, he helped me see that too. He's since become a mentor and supporter in this next chapter: gently nudging, believing, cheering me on, and reminding me that my voice is needed now, not later.

There's never going to be a perfect time to write this book. Cool Beans will keep growing. Life will keep moving. But this story – my story – needs to be told now. Not just for me. Not just for Cool Beans. But for everyone who needs to hear what's at stake when it comes to men's health. Because this is bigger than my fertility story. It's a window into something larger – the health of men everywhere, and the impact that has on everyone.

So here I am. Writing my first book. No ghostwriter. No filter. Just a hell of a story, a mission that matters, and Andrew now firmly in my corner. What you'll find in these pages isn't polished perfection. It's lived experience. It's truth. It's mine.

You'll also come across additional sections called This Side of the Story throughout the book – just like this one. These are real-time reflections I've written while working on the book. Moments of pause. Honest thoughts. Sometimes messy. Often revealing. They're here to bring you closer to where I am now, as I look back and write forward.

If you've picked up this book, maybe you already sense that something needs to change. You're right. And I'm glad you're here. Let's dive in.

# FOREWORD

There are books that entertain, others that inform, and then there are ones like COOL BEANS that hold a mirror to your own life and quietly, powerfully, change you. Saara Jamison has written something rare, a book that doesn't just ask to be read, but invites you into a journey that is as much yours as it is hers. You reflect on your journey, your friend's journey, your family's journey and more importantly your future.

When conversations around fertility, hormone regulation, and miscarriages arise, the focus is almost always on women. It's where the spotlight has sat for decades, where the bulk of medical research, treatment, and social awareness have been directed and yet, very few people acknowledge, let alone truly consider, the role of men's reproductive health. What about the impact of stress, poor sleep, poor nutrition, or testicular heat on sperm quality? What about the silence so many men carry when their partners are hurting? What about the very real neglect of male bodies in this conversation? I'm guilty of this myself and I consider myself an educated health professional.

This is where COOL BEANS steps in, with the missing piece of the reproductive puzzle. It's a thought-provoking account that combines lived experience with the science needed to satisfy even the most analytical reader. Saara sheds light on an aspect of reproductive wellbeing that has been overlooked for too long, reminding us that fertility is not just a woman's story. It is a human story. By bringing men back into the fertility conversation, she challenges outdated narratives and opens the door to a more complete, balanced understanding of reproductive health.

When I was first asked to support Saara Jamison in her mission to improve men's health, I was honoured. But it wasn't until I sat down and read her book that I truly understood the depth of her passion and felt compelled to help her share it with the world. As a recent author myself, with *Blokes Inc. Play a Bigger Game*, I know firsthand what it takes to pour your heart, your research, and your lived experience into a manuscript. I also know the responsibility that comes with daring to speak on issues that many shy away from. For me, the "perfect threesome": sleep hygiene, nutrition, and exercise, form the foundation for optimal performance and wellbeing. These are the pillars I return to again and again in my own work.

What struck me most about *COOL BEANS* was how it follows a similar threesome formula, but in a space where the conversation has been almost silent. Instead of sleep, nutrition, and exercise, Saara shines a light on testicular heat, the collapse of male health, and the neglect of male bodies. Her framework is practical, compelling, and refreshingly honest. Saara's passion is not only evident in the pages of this book; it radiates from her mission. She provides hope where there has been despair, clarity where there has been confusion, and perhaps most importantly, reassurance for those who may feel alone in their fertility journey.

Together, our approaches as new authors complement and strengthen one another. Where my work urges men to play a bigger game with their health and performance, becoming proactive rather than reactive, Saara's reminds us that the stakes are not just personal; they are generational. When passion and purpose align, the impact on men's health can be truly transformative.

# Foreword

This book doesn't shy away from the difficult parts. It walks unflinchingly through the realities of fertility struggles, the quiet ache of waiting, the societal silence around men's reproductive health, and the recognition that love alone is not always enough; yet, in these moments, COOL BEANS never loses its thread of hope.

What makes this story extraordinary is how beautifully it blends vulnerability with strength. You'll find science here, practical, evidence-based insights about fertility, nutrition, testicular health, and preconception care. What I also love is Saara's journey and her lived experiences of a couple navigating the unknown. It is this balance of emotion and information that makes COOL BEANS uniquely compelling.

Too often, books about fertility lean to one extreme: either they drown you in cold statistics or they offer personal stories without context or depth. Saara balances both perfectly, and in doing so, she creates a narrative that feels both relatable and reliable.

COOL BEANS cleverly keeps you engaged from start to finish. Each chapter doesn't just deliver knowledge; it follows through with a practical section called 'Putting it into practice'. Here, readers are given simple, actionable steps that can be taken immediately.

This structure makes the book far more than just information; it is a tool for transformation. Whether it's steps you can take on your own, strategies you can share with your partner, or changes you can make together, this format ensures that every reader feels empowered to apply what they've just learned. It's engaging, interactive, and accessible, bridging the gap between awareness and action. Let's be honest: as a male in the health and wellness industry, I know first-hand that men's health conversations desperately need more of that.

Books like this matter because they connect. They offer insight, but they also extend a hand. Whether you're just beginning your own fertility journey, supporting a partner through it, or reflecting on the winding road you've already walked, COOL BEANS offers connection. It offers perspective. And most of all, it offers hope.

Saara's writing makes you feel seen, understood, and less alone. You'll laugh at moments, perhaps cry at others, but you will always feel the steady undercurrent of encouragement. This is not a book written to lecture or shame you; it is written to guide you and remind you that, even in the face of difficulty, there is always a way forward. Isn't that what we all need in the end? Hope. The belief that change is possible. The comfort of knowing that we're not alone.

Unfortunately, we live in an age where men's health is collapsing under the weight of poor lifestyle choices, relentless stress, and the myths of masculinity that keep men silent. Sperm counts are declining globally. Male infertility is on the rise and yet, so much of the conversation still assumes fertility is a woman's issue. *COOL BEANS* dismantles that myth with clarity and compassion, and for this I love it. It reminds us that reproductive health is shared health. That men's choices, environments, and habits matter deeply, not just for themselves, but for their partners, their families, and more importantly, their future children. By bringing this conversation into the light, Saara not only raises awareness but also empowers action, which is exactly what makes this book so necessary, so relevant, and so urgent right now.

As I turned the pages of *COOL BEANS*, I found myself reflecting on my own work and the many men I've coached, trained, and supported over the years. Men who've battled addiction. Men who've struggled with anxiety and depression. Men who've pushed so hard in their careers that their health and their families suffered as a result.

Time and again, the same truth reveals itself: when men neglect their health, the impact ripples far beyond themselves. It touches their partners, their children, their communities. The same is true for fertility. It is not just about one person's biology, it is about shared wellbeing, shared choices and shared futures. That is why I find this book so moving and so necessary. It's not just about sperm counts or testicular heat. It's about men stepping back into the conversation, not as silent

# Foreword

bystanders, but as active participants in their own health and their shared journey toward family.

Saara has given us a gift with *COOL BEANS*. She has taken a topic many shy away from and approached it with honesty, courage, and compassion. She has woven science with story, data with dialogue, and in doing so, created something that speaks both to the head and the heart. For men, this book is a wake-up call. For women, it is a window into a side of the fertility conversation that is often left unspoken. For couples, it is an opportunity to walk this road together, with greater understanding, clarity, and connection.

As you turn these pages, I invite you to do so with an open heart and an open mind. Let yourself be challenged. Let yourself be moved. Let yourself be changed, because *COOL BEANS* is not just a book you read and put back on the shelf. It is a book that stays with you. It is a book that sparks conversations, inspires action, and, if you let it, changes the way you see your own health and your role in the bigger picture of fertility and family.

You're about to walk alongside a story that will make you laugh, maybe cry, and most certainly think. For those of you who have been on this journey, or are now on this journey, you'll feel seen, understood, and empowered. Perhaps, like Saara herself, you'll find yourself inspired to share your story too…

This is more than a book. It is a movement, and I, for one, am honoured to be walking alongside it.

HELP ONE: HELP MANY

**Tory Trewhitt**
Author of *Blokes Inc. Play a Bigger Game*

**CoolBeans**

## PROLOGUE
# WHERE WE ARE TODAY

Today, Cool Beans has moved from our kitchen table to the wider world. We've been recognised on national stages and in the media – double winner at River Rival Pitch competition (People's Choice & Best Product), Queensland 40Under40 and Game Changer winner, ORIAS Small Business Innovation winner, Startup World Cup QLD finalist, iAwards national finalist – and featured everywhere from the Today Show to the Sydney Morning Herald, as well as Brisbane's MedTech Global Accelerator "fast lane" list. These aren't just trophies; they're signals that men's health is finally being taken seriously – and that a simple, science-led idea can shift how families plan, recover and thrive.

Clinicians, athletes and everyday families are now using Cool Beans as a practical, stigma-free way to reduce heat and support fertility, hormone balance and recovery – a small change with compounding benefits for couples and future kids.

Why me? You might wonder why I, Saara – a daughter, wife, sister, mother, aunt, and founder of Cool Beans – am leading the conversation on men's health. I am surrounded by men whose lives shape mine and the lives of everyone I love. Health is not a solitary thing – it ripples out. It touches every part of how we – and those around us – live, love, and dream. Without our health, we have nothing. And when men's health is neglected, families and futures suffer too.

I'm writing this from our veranda on thirty acres west of Brisbane, watching Jordan, my husband, play with our two children. Their laughter mingles with our dogs' excited barks as they chase the chickens – twenty-odd of them – and six ducks around the yard. Every day, there's a new discussion – whether goats or cows or pigs should be next on our little homestead – today, it's goats.

We've built a home that's full of love and adventure. A place where we have open conversations around a fire, listen to audiobooks, learn to read and now to play guitar too. My children, Van and Heidi, are eight and six. For all the things I've done in my life, nothing makes me prouder than raising these two, shaping them into the people they're becoming.

You'll also hear directly from Jordan in his own chapter. His experience, and the decisions he made along the way, were central to how this journey unfolded. While this book is largely told from my perspective, his contribution matters deeply. It's his story too, and his voice belongs in this conversation just as much as mine.

But the path I'm on now isn't one I wrote for myself. It was forged by years of struggle, heartbreak, and finally a joy so big I can't explain it – followed by the heavy weight of too much knowledge.

When I look at our children's future, I see troubling trends. Men's health is declining across the board – physical, mental and reproductive health all on the wane – and with it, the wellbeing of our children. More babies arrive today facing challenges my generation rarely saw. I don't want Van or Heidi to step out into this world fearful of the battles their parents faced. I don't want them daunted by fertility struggles or ashamed of whatever path leads them to conception – whether it's natural, IVF (In Vitro Fertilisation), surrogacy, adoption or donation.

## Prologue: Where we are today

I've walked that road myself: miscarriages and failed attempts that tested our marriage and our faith in what was possible. Assisted reproduction shines brightest when it's the last step, not the first. Build your foundation with everyday habits, nourishing meals, stress breaks, proper rest and scrotal cooling, and you'll enter the clinic as your own strongest fertility protocol.

Too many men still carry their struggles quietly. That silence helps explain why suicide rates continue to raise and why chronic conditions are often picked up late. In fertility care, we sometimes move straight to treatment before laying the groundwork – simple, powerful steps like a semen analysis, and addressing factors like sleep and nutrition, movement and weight, heat exposure, alcohol and medications, and stress, for both women and men. What IVF has been able to do today is mind-blowing, and for many families, essential; though too few lay the groundwork and improve health fundamentals before pursuing it. I'm speaking up because my kids are watching, and because my goal is bigger than our family: a community ethos that makes caring for men's health simple, shared, and stigma-free.

This is why it matters that I, a woman, am leading this charge. I'm not here to tiptoe around awkward conversations or worry about making people uncomfortable. Men's health matters for all of us, and it's time to break the silence. If I don't do this, who will? My children are counting on me, but it's not enough to help only them. This fight is bigger than just us – it's about building a healthier world for everyone.

Every family matters equally, whether single parents, same-sex partners, adopting, fostering, or blended. This book is for everyone who believes in building healthier families and stronger generations.

Cool Beans Underwear® began as a small idea to help Jordan and me conceive. It's now a mission: advocacy for men's health without shame, grounded in evidence and lived experience. Being a mother gave me purpose; being an advocate gives that purpose a voice.

Being a mother drives me forward, but being an advocate gives purpose to that drive. My children and my partner fuel this mission, but so does the belief that we deserve a world where men can care for their health without shame or silence.

I'm sharing my story not just for me, but for you – whether you're a partner, a parent, or someone who simply believes in a healthier future. My hope is that in these pages you find reasons to care, to speak up and to join me in building a stronger next generation.

Before I could build this mission, I had to live it. Let me take you back to where it all began.

If any part of you feels this isn't your story, that fertility is someone else's burden, or that prevention is out of reach, I invite you to stay open. What changed our lives started with one uncomfortable question, one unexpected solution, and one moment of honesty. That's how this all began.

I hope this story inspires you to be part of this change. Because if we want to secure the future for our children and their children, it starts with us – today.

## Putting it into practice

**For him** – Small habits today protect your fertility tomorrow.

- Cool your crown jewels:
    - Wear loose-fitting, breathable underwear designed to reduce scrotal heat.
    - Even small increases in scrotal temperature reduce sperm count and motility.
    - Men who lowered scrotal temperature by 1°C saw a 49% increase in sperm concentration (Jung et al., 2005).

- Exercise smart – not overheated:
  - Choose moderate-intensity exercise (walking, swimming, weights) for 30 minutes a day. Avoid prolonged cycling or HIIT (High Intensity Interval Training) daily.
  - Movement improves hormone balance and reduces oxidative stress, but overheating can do more harm than good.
  - Moderate exercise improves sperm quality; intense training can suppress reproductive hormones (Vaamonde et al., 2012).
- Feed your fertility:
  - Eat a diet rich in vegetables, healthy fats, whole grains, and zinc (nuts, seeds, shellfish).
  - Diet is a direct input into sperm health; processed foods and alcohol are linked to DNA damage.
  - A healthy diet improves sperm motility and morphology (Chavarro et al., 2007).

**For her** – Your health influences every part of this journey.

- Reset your stress hormones:
  - Commit to 10 minutes of daily mindfulness, breathwork or guided meditation.
  - Cortisol and adrenaline interfere with reproductive hormone function, even low-level daily stress adds up.
  - Women in IVF programs who practised mindfulness had improved emotional wellbeing and higher pregnancy rates (Galhardo et al., 2013).
- Nourish with intention:
  - Prioritise whole foods, especially leafy greens, healthy fats, and plant-based iron sources like legumes and pumpkin seeds.
  - Nutrient deficiencies disrupt ovulation, hormone balance, and implantation.
  - Diets rich in folate, iron and healthy fats increase chances of conception (Chavarro et al., 2007).

- Start the sperm talk early:
  - Don't wait to talk about male fertility, even before trying to conceive; get a sperm analysis done.
  - Male-factor infertility accounts for 40-50% of infertility cases, but is often ignored until late in the process (Agarwal et al., 2015).

**For us** – Connection is as vital as conception.

- Talk before you try:
  - Schedule a weekly check-in that goes beyond to-do lists. Ask: "How are we coping, really?"
  - Stress, resentment and unspoken fears erode connection and can impact fertility outcomes.
  - Couples who maintain emotional closeness during fertility challenges report higher satisfaction and lower distress (Peterson et al., 2006).
- Create joy, not just goals:
  - Plan one shared experience each week: a movie, a meal, a slow walk – no fertility talk allowed.
  - Fun buffers stress and reminds couples that their relationship is more than a reproductive mission.
  - Shared leisure activities significantly improve relationship resilience (Wise et al., 2012).
- Choose a team mentality:
  - Frame fertility as a "we" issue from day one, not just hers to solve or his to fix.
  - Shared responsibility improves communication and reduces shame or blame.
  - Couples who view infertility as a shared challenge report stronger relationship outcomes (Galst, 2010).

Prologue: Where we are today

## Behind the chapter: Sources

- Moderate exercise improves sperm parameters and hormone balance (Vaamonde et al., 2012).
- Scrotal cooling improves sperm count and motility (Jung et al., 2005).
- Diet and micronutrients are directly tied to reproductive health in both sexes (Chavarro et al., 2007).
- Mindfulness improves resilience and pregnancy rates during fertility treatment (Galhardo et al., 2013).
- Emotional connection improves fertility outcomes (Peterson et al., 2006).
- Male factor infertility is present in 40-50% of cases (Agarwal et al., 2015).

**CoolBeans**

## PREFACE
# THE DAY I KNEW

I wasn't one to rush in when it came to love – until I met Jordan, whose kindness and shared sense of adventure changed everything. Prior to that, my longest relationship had lasted over three years, starting when I was just twenty. In 2010, I left everything behind and moved to Africa for a gap year. I trained as a Big Five animal field guide, taking people on game walks and drives. It was one of the best years of my life – living in a world so different to home, one filled with beauty and danger, with animals that could not only kill you, but eat you too. The thought of being someone's prey was never far from my mind.

That year in Africa taught me so much about myself. It taught me how to be brave, how to embrace the unknown, and how to find my way through fear and doubt. When I came back home, I brought that spirit with me. I wanted that same sense of purpose and adventure in my relationships, but I found myself falling into the same old patterns.

I dated another man when I got back, but it was more of the same. Meeting men had never been the problem – finding the right one was the challenge. They were usually older, different, never one I could see a future with. I was always trying to make it work, even when it didn't feel right.

By 2012, I'd decided enough was enough. I wanted to meet someone closer to my age, someone who shared my dreams and who felt like home. So, I turned to online dating. It was a leap for me, but I was ready for something real.

I only ever spoke to one man online. Jordan. We could talk for hours, even before we met. Our conversations flowed so easily, like I'd known him forever. Jordan was only three years older than me, close enough in age that we shared a similar outlook on life. On the 26th of May 2012, we finally met in-person at a bar in Brisbane. I was living too far out of the city, so I'd planned to stay at a girlfriend's place – as it turned out, I didn't need somewhere else to stay that night.

The moment I saw Jordan, I felt a spark I hadn't felt before. He was tall, taller than me even when I was in heels – and I'm not short. I leaned in and gave him a cuddle and a kiss on the cheek while he tried to shake my hand. He was nervous, I could see; a little awkward, but so genuine. Meeting someone in-person for the first time is always a bit strange – do you shake hands, hug, kiss? Me, I'm a cuddler and a kisser; and, as it turned out, so was Jordan.

The date was perfect. My girlfriend was hosting a party for a friend's birthday at another bar, so we crashed it. Everything felt so easy, like I'd known him for years. I felt no awkwardness, no hesitation. My walls were down, and I could see myself with this man. He made me feel safe, like he would always have my back – and oh, hasn't he proven that to me over the years.

By July we had moved in together into a private little 80s-style unit, down four flights of stairs, with our own garden and courtyard in Brisbane city. I loved that unit. We had some ups and downs in the early days. We were still figuring each other out, learning to trust and communicate. What I learned from those challenges was that my instinct was right – Jordan would always have my back. If we could get through those tough moments and come out stronger, I knew he was the one for me. I had no doubt.

## Preface: The day I knew

I didn't always feel like I deserved this man. I was still young at 26, still learning how to be true to myself. I'd always been a people-pleaser, someone who didn't want to disappoint or cause conflict. It had made me easy to manipulate, and in the end, it always hurt someone. But if Jordan could forgive me for my mistakes, if he could see the real me and still want to be with me, then nothing was going to stand in my way of building a life with him. I knew he would be the best husband and an even better father. I guess I scared him too, but even through the hurt, he could see what we had, and he wanted to hold onto that too.

By October we were engaged, and by March married – Easter Saturday 2013.

It is still the best wedding I have ever been to. There was so much fun to be had. We got married at my brother's farm at Maleny which, through word of mouth, kept getting booked for weddings after ours and eventually became The Old Dairy Wedding Venue. Now that it's a commercial business, it's gorgeous and wins plenty of awards. It's still unique, but it doesn't quite have what we had. A marquee wedding with hay bales, open fields, and cows peeking in to see what we were up to. It was magical. It was fun. There was not a single issue, other than getting a text message from my future mother-in-law on the morning of the wedding, saying that Jordan had never made it home the night before. All the boys had gone out early for a few drinks which turned into a massive night including mischievous antics (like snorting tobacco). I don't blame Jordan – he was out with my older brothers, and I have no doubt they were leading the charge.

It had rained all day on the day of our wedding. But as I got into the car to drive there, the clouds parted, and it stopped raining – which made for the most majestic photography, with storm clouds still rolling around.

The following day – Easter Sunday – everyone was welcomed back for a barbecue breakfast, leftover champagne, and my husband sporting the most obscure outfit as he had misplaced his bag. But he was my man and boy, didn't I love him. At that time, I didn't think it possible to love him or anybody more, but as it turned out, that's probably when I loved him the least. He has gone on to be the amazing husband and dad I knew he would be. And now, 12 years of marriage later, I still say I don't think I could possibly love him any more than I do now. I can't wait to see where this love grows to in the next 12 years.

After our wedding, we honeymooned in Phuket and Phi Phi Island, where we continued to discuss planning for our family. It was here in Thailand that we began our conception journey, struggling to keep our hands off each other and starting to try for our baby. I now appreciate that this journey looks different for every family – whether natural, IVF, surrogacy, adoption or donation – and it's precisely why preparing your health first matters so much.

We were blissfully unaware of what was coming. At that time, fertility was just a concept, not a diagnosis. We thought love was enough. But as I now know, preparing your body and mind for parenthood is about more than timing and romance. It's biology. It's lifestyle. It's health. And for men, it's a health crisis hiding in plain sight.

We were young and in love. At the time, it felt like there was nothing in the world that could stop us. Looking back now, I see how naive we were, how we thought that if you loved someone enough, that was all it took. But even in those early days, there was so much hope, so much joy, and so much belief in the future we were building together. Little did we know that that future would be tested in ways we never imagined. And that's where this story really begins.

*Preface: The day I knew*

## Putting it into practice

**For him** – Support sperm health through simple lifestyle shifts.

- Limit alcohol to protect sperm quality:
  o Cap intake at 2 standard drinks per week.
  o Alcohol is directly linked to decreased sperm count, motility, and morphology.
  o Even moderate drinking has been associated with altered reproductive hormones and semen quality (Tønnesen et al., 2014).
- Hydrate like your fertility depends on it:
  o Drink at least 2 litres of water daily.
  o Staying hydrated supports testosterone production and maintains healthy semen volume.
  o Dehydration disrupts hormone function and reduces ejaculate volume (Popkin et al., 2010).

**For her** – Consume antioxidants and alkalinity for reproductive vitality.

- Load up on antioxidant-rich foods:
  o Include at least 5 servings of brightly coloured fruits and vegetables each day.
  o These combat oxidative stress, which damages eggs and impacts fertility.
  o Antioxidant intake has been linked with improved egg quality and pregnancy rates (Agarwal et al., 2014).
- Alkalise your body gently with lemon water:
  o Add fresh lemon juice to your water in the morning.
    - 'Alkalising' = even though lemon juice is acidic in the glass, after digestion it has an alkaline effect (lowers your diet's acid load). This shows up mostly in urine and doesn't change blood pH.

- Alkalising foods may support cervical mucus quality and uterine health.
- Diets with high antioxidant and alkalising foods are associated with improved conception outcomes (Vujkovic et al., 2010).

**For us** – Build a healthy foundation together.

- Move your bodies – and your bond:
  - Plan a shared outdoor activity once a week (walk, hike, bike).
  - Joint physical activity reduces stress, strengthens connection, and improves metabolic markers.
  - Couples who exercise together report stronger relationships and reduced fertility-related stress (Wise et al., 2012).
- Unwind as a daily ritual, not just as a reward:
  - Create a calming evening routine: herbal tea, 10 minutes of yoga or stretching, and screen-free time.
  - Good sleep and reduced cortisol support reproductive hormones for both partners.
  - Evening wind-down routines improve sleep quality and emotional regulation (Pien & Schwab, 2004).

## Behind the chapter: Sources

- Alcohol shows a dose–response association with poorer semen quality and altered reproductive hormones, even at modest weekly intake (Jensen et al., 2014).
- Antioxidant strategies in fertility/ART contexts may support reproductive outcomes; evidence varies by context (Agarwal et al., 2014).
- A preconception Mediterranean-style diet has been associated with higher IVF/ICSI pregnancy rates (Vujkovic et al., 2010).

- Physical activity: moderate is generally helpful; high volumes of vigorous activity can delay conception in normal-BMI women (Wise et al., 2012).
- Sleep: one week of short sleep reduces testosterone in healthy young men; protect sleep to support hormones (Leproult & Van Cauter, 2011).
- Hydration: adequate water intake supports overall physiological function and fluid balance, including semen volume (Popkin et al., 2010).

**CoolBeans**

# PART I

## STARTING THE JOURNEY

**CoolBeans**

# CHAPTER 1
# THE WONDER OF WHAT COULD BE

Those two years after our wedding felt like a dream, even though the baby we hoped for still hadn't come. We were young and in love, sure that our future would unfold just as we imagined. Yet beneath that joy, I sensed something darker: men's health everywhere was slipping – physical fitness, mental wellbeing and reproductive strength alike – and I was determined our family would be the exception.

When we moved back home to the family property west of Brisbane, it wasn't the bustling farm of my childhood anymore. My parents had retired and moved north to Bundaberg, leaving behind the old house filled with the memories and clutter of our family. My brothers still dropped by, wandering in like they always had, and at first, Jordan and I felt a little lost within those walls – as if we were visitors in someone else's story.

I grew up in that house. My brothers were 11 and 14 years older than me – not exactly ideal playmates. Luckily, our neighbours were like a second family. They had four incredible kids who became the siblings I didn't have at home – and still are today.

They helped raise me. They exposed me to the wild, chaotic joy of childhood freedom: the kind where you've got land to roam, imaginations to run with, and just enough stupidity to think your dumbest ideas are brilliant. We shot arrows straight into the sky. We did donuts in our bush-basher – with someone clinging to the roof. We should have broken bones, or worse. But somehow, we made it through, mostly unscathed.

In between the chaos, we built cubbies in trees and lean-tos deep in the gullies. We hiked to the river in the reserve across the road, spent whole days fishing, exploring, getting dirty, getting sunburnt. No adults hovered – it was just fresh air, sunshine and the resilience that comes from true freedom. I'd come to see how those early choices – outdoor play, fresh food, risk and recovery – are exactly the building blocks of long-term health.

We were lucky – not every kid gets a childhood like that. We grew up on a property, with hundreds of acres of nature reserve across the road as our backyard. And I had my neighbours to thank for making that life not just possible, but magical. They filled my childhood with adventure, gave me laughter, gave me freedom, and gave me a full heart.

All I ever wanted was to raise my kids here too – to give them what I had. That wild and free kind of childhood that so many children today never get to taste.

Back to when Jordan and I moved into my family home – over the next year, we made that space ours. We decluttered, repaired, and rebuilt. We turned the property into a small, working homestead with chickens and pigs, and even a couple of sheep and goats. I loved the idea of self-sufficiency; of caring for what went into my body and the home I was creating. I started a vegetable garden, and together with Jordan, we raised and processed our own animals. We had all the fresh vegetables and meat we could ask for. We had everything we'd dreamed of – except the one thing we wanted most. Month after month passed in hopeful silence, until hope began to feel like something heavier: uncertainty.

All of our friends were starting families; our siblings too – they made it look so easy. Only one friend that I knew of struggled and they were also a family member – losing their first child before going on to have two beautiful boys. Back then, I didn't fully understand that kind of heartbreak, but I carried a quiet ache inside me – a longing that grew with every new pregnancy announcement.

Yet, I came to realise every family's path is unique, not just here in Australia, but globally. Whether natural, IVF, adoption, or surrogacy, struggles are shared universally. From Sydney to San Francisco, infertility affects millions, connecting us all in an invisible yet profound way.

What unites all of us, regardless of how our families are formed, is the need for knowledge, preparation, and care. Fertility isn't just a woman's burden. And too often, men are left out of the conversation entirely.

Still, life was good. We were fit and strong, lifting weights and training for triathlons. I've always loved hiking, but there's something different about multi-day treks – carrying everything you need, relying only on yourself and the person beside you. Those trips were about adventure, but also about peace. They were about finding ourselves in the wilderness and feeling alive in a way that only the unknown can bring.

Those years weren't just about waiting for a baby. They were about learning who we were together. They were about building a home that felt like ours, a life that felt like ours. We travelled and explored, always with that quiet ache, but also with a deep joy in the life we were creating.

On our first multi-day trek along the Sunshine Coast Great Walk – we hadn't trained – we had no idea what to pack, which also meant our backpacks were way too heavy. The trail wound through the hinterland, up and down, up and down, for four days. It was brutal. But we were in it together.

And that's what made it so powerful. We had space to just be – no distractions, no deadlines, no grief tugging at us from the corners of our minds. Just us, walking side by side. We'd already been through so much, and this gave us a chance to reconnect, to feel like a team again.

At the end of the hike, we booked one night at a Bed & Breakfast tucked away on a remote property outside of Maleny. There was champagne waiting, a hot tub, and a sunset over the mountains. That night gave us a rare kind of peace – an escape from the heartbreak of home. A pause to breathe. To sit in the stillness and soak in the love we still had for each other. To remember that even in the chaos of grief and loss, we still had this: us.

Looking back now, I see how much those years gave us. They taught us that life isn't just about what comes next – it's about how we show up for each other, even in the waiting. They taught us that health and love are built in the small, everyday choices – in the food we grew, the animals we raised, the laughter around the dinner table.

There was so much hope, so much belief in the future we were building. And that hope, that belief – it carried us through everything.

I didn't know then that these sweet, quiet years would be the last of our innocence. But I can see now that they gave us the strength we'd need when the path grew harder. They gave us something to hold onto – the memory of who we were, and who we could be, together.

## Putting it into practice

**For him** – Build hormonal strength from the plate up.

- Prioritise whole, unprocessed meals:
    - Prepare a homemade lunch each day using whole foods.
    - Reduce exposure to preservatives and processed additives that interfere with testosterone and sperm production.
    - Men who consume more home-cooked meals have better semen quality and hormonal balance (Mendoza et al., 2017).
- Cut back on sugary drinks:
    - Replace sodas and energy drinks with water or herbal tea.
    - Excess sugar intake is linked to reduced testosterone and sperm motility.
    - Just one sugary drink per day is associated with reduced fertility in men and women (Chiu et al., 2014).

**For her** – Nourish your cycle with hydration and enzymes.

- Stay consistently hydrated:
    - Drink 2–3 litres of water daily.
    - Supports cervical mucus production and hormonal regulation.
    - Hydration improves reproductive function and hormone transport (Popkin et al., 2010).
- Harness the power of pineapple:
    - Eat fresh pineapple core during your two-week wait.
        - Two-week wait = the ~14 days between ovulation/embryo transfer and your pregnancy test.
    - Contains bromelain, which may support implantation through improved blood flow.
    - Bromelain has mild anticoagulant and anti-inflammatory properties potentially beneficial in early conception (Kline, 2017).

**For us** – Make food a ritual of connection.

- Cook together, grow together:
  - Try one new healthy recipe together each week.
  - Joint food preparation boosts emotional intimacy and healthy eating habits.
  - Couples who cook together report better diet quality and stronger relationship satisfaction (Hammiche et al., 2012).
- Protect shared mealtimes:
  - Sit down together for meals without screens or distractions.
  - Increases bonding, improves digestion and mindful eating.
  - Families that eat together regularly show stronger cohesion and better nutrition outcomes (Fiese et al., 2012).

**For all families** – Honour every path to parenthood.

- Learn your landscape early:
  - Research IVF, IUI (Intrauterine Insemination), surrogacy, adoption and donor options available in your region.
  - Reduces fear and stigma by replacing unknowns with informed decisions.
  - Access to early fertility education improves mental health and planning outcomes (Hammarberg et al., 2017).
- Find your community:
  - Join an inclusive fertility support group (online or in-person).
  - Sharing the journey with others reduces stress and improves emotional resilience.
  - Social support improves IVF success and psychological wellbeing during fertility treatment (Greil et al., 2011).

## Behind the Chapter: Sources

- Processed food intake is linked to hormonal disruption and lower fertility in men and women (Mendoza et al., 2017).
- Even mild dehydration interferes with reproductive hormone balance and mucus production (Popkin et al., 2010).
- Sugar-sweetened beverages are associated with decreased fertility across both sexes (Chiu et al., 2014).
- Couples who share meals and co-cook report stronger relationship satisfaction and better nutritional choices (Hammiche et al., 2012; Fiese et al., 2012).
- High stress and depressive symptoms in men predict up to a 30% greater risk of chronic disease by age 50 (Aitken et al., 2019).

**CoolBeans**

## CHAPTER 2

# THE DAY THE LINE FADED

I had always imagined the day I'd see those two pink lines. When it finally happened, it felt like the world had stopped just for me. That moment means so much – whether you're trying naturally, pursuing IVF, surrogacy, adoption or egg/sperm donation – each of us holds our own hopes in that tiny plastic stick.

Jordan was still asleep when I took the test. I knew his joy would match mine – though I also felt the familiar stirring of worry for him, because too often men bear the hidden weight of fertility stress. The first pink line appeared immediately, then the wait – the longest minutes of my life. And then there it was – the second line, faint at first but growing stronger. My hands were shaking as I stared at it, the proof of the life growing inside me.

I did a little dance on the spot, punching the air with the test in my hand, unable to contain the joy that was bursting from my chest. I walked out of the bathroom, sat down beside Jordan, and placed the test on his bedside table.

I kissed him on the forehead and waited. "Good morning, sweetheart," he murmured, brushing a strand of hair from my face.

Jordan always had a way of penetrating my soul and seeing what was there – as I did him. He never made me doubt or feel unloved. He was special like that, always ensuring I felt safe, seen, and wanted.

The look in his eyes that morning was no different – soft and sure – and I remember wondering how that love might shift when we had a child. I know now: it didn't shift. It only grew.

I didn't say anything – just held up the test, my grin so wide it felt like it might split my face.

He sat up, took the test from my hands, his eyes wide with wonder. "Are you really… are we…?"

"Yes," I whispered. "You're going to be a dad."

He wrapped me in his arms, kissing me all over, his hands gently resting on my belly. We were giddy with hope, already imagining the life we were about to build.

Two months later, it was my 29th birthday. Jordan treated me like a queen. He made me breakfast – toast, tea, my favourite jam. We curled up on the couch, wrapped in the glow of that new life. We laughed and talked about names – even the silly ones we'd never use. For a little while, it felt like everything was exactly as it should be.

Then, while I was enjoying my second cup of tea, I felt a small cramp low in my belly. It caught me off guard, but I brushed it aside. Early pregnancy has so many strange sensations, I told myself. But when I went to the bathroom, I saw the first streak of bright red. My breath caught in my chest, and the world around me seemed to stop.

I walked back into the living room, my face carefully controlled. Jordan looked up from where he sat on the couch, his smile fading immediately. "I'm bleeding," I said quietly.

He pulled me close and held me, his arms strong and steady around me. "It could be nothing, sweetheart," he said, his voice gentle but edged with worry. "Spotting can be normal. Let's not panic yet."

But I could see it in his eyes – the same fear I felt deep in my own chest. He called the doctor straight away, his voice calm even as his hands shook just a little. The receptionist told him to bring me in for blood tests right away.

He offered to stay home from work, but I shook my head. "There's nothing you can do here," I said, though a part of me wanted him to stay, to hold me through the waiting.

He kissed me on the forehead, his thumb brushing the tears from my cheeks. "It's going to be okay," he said. "It might just be a scare." He said the words for me, even though I could tell he wasn't sure if he believed them.

Then he was gone, off to work, and I was left to drive to the clinic alone, the fear sitting like a stone in my chest. The drive felt endless – every stoplight, every turn, every second was filled with a dread that made it hard to breathe.

The waiting room was a blur. I sat there, clutching my phone, every buzz making my heart leap. The blood test was quick, but the wait for the results felt like an eternity. They promised they'd call me as soon as they had them, but the hours dragged on.

When I got home, the house was so quiet. My birthday gifts sat unopened on the counter. The messages from friends and family wishing me a happy birthday felt like they belonged to someone else. My phone stayed glued to my hand, but the call never came.

Jordan came home that evening and put his arms around me, stroking my belly – silently. We didn't talk much – what was there to say? We went to bed that night still with no word from the doctor, even though the bloods were marked as urgent. The silence was deafening.

At 11:26pm, my phone buzzed on the nightstand. My heart leapt, hoping for good news – but as soon as I saw the message, my heart shattered. My GP's words were blunt and clinical: "I'm sorry. This pregnancy isn't going to last. Please call me tomorrow so we can plan next steps."

It felt like the air had been punched out of my lungs. My chest tightened, and I began to cry, the tears coming hard and fast, my breath catching in jagged gasps. I was hyperventilating, my whole body shaking – Jordan wrapped me in his arms, silent tears running down his cheeks too. He never asked me to stop crying, he never asked me to calm down. He just held me, his arms strong around me, grounding me in that moment of heartbreak.

He was breaking too, but he was my rock. He held me until there was nothing left in me, until the tears finally slowed, and exhaustion pulled me under. We fell asleep like that – him holding me, my head on his chest, the two of us wrapped in a grief so heavy it felt like it might swallow us whole.

The next day, the bleeding began in earnest. It was no longer just spotting – it was like a floodgate had opened. The blood came thick and clotted, full of tissue and mucous, so different from any regular period. My cramps grew sharper, more insistent, radiating through my back and belly. My body felt swollen and tender, my head pounding with grief.

I couldn't use a tampon – I needed the biggest pad I could find, something to hold back the tide. I felt dizzy from the blood loss, lightheaded every time I stood. My body felt like it was betraying me, letting go of something I'd only just begun to love.

We're told not to talk about pregnancy in those first twelve weeks, as if silence can protect us from the pain if it all falls apart. But that silence only made me feel more alone.

Yet, I wasn't alone. Globally, one in four pregnancies end in miscarriage. Millions silently grieve, each believing they're alone. This isn't just my story, or an Australian story; it's a global story. Yet despite its prevalence, so many of us are told to stay silent, to wait until we've "made it through the first trimester" before we share. But when the loss comes, silence doesn't protect us, it isolates us.

The day after I lost the baby, I walked next door to my sister-in-law's house. She had been through it too – she knew what this pain felt like. She was feeding her little boy in his highchair when I walked in. "I miscarried," I said, my voice breaking. "I've lost my baby." She stood up and pulled me close. I sobbed into her shoulder, and she just held me. She didn't try to fix it. She didn't offer empty words. She just held me – and in that moment, I didn't feel so alone.

That moment showed me the power of community – whether you're a straight couple, same-sex partners, a solo parent or in another family form, none of us should grieve alone.

What if we approached early pregnancy with the same openness we offer in other parts of life? What if we talked about the highs *and* the heartbreaks? Grief doesn't grow smaller in the dark, but it softens in the presence of others.

That first miscarriage changed me. It was the day my life imploded – the day everything shifted. My birthday will always carry the weight of that loss, but it also marks the day I started to understand just how strong I could be.

I didn't know it then, but this loss would become the cornerstone of something bigger, a mission to ensure other families didn't have to walk through this alone, and that men's and women's reproductive health would stop being hidden in silence and shame. The grief that cracked me open was also what lit the first spark of a mission I never could have imagined. And that's what the next chapter is about.

## Putting it into practice

**For him** – Protect reproductive health through stress management and movement.

- Manage stress to protect sperm health:
  - Dedicate 10–15 minutes daily to breathwork, meditation, or mindfulness.
  - Chronic stress disrupts testosterone and impairs sperm production.
  - Men with high perceived stress have significantly lower sperm concentration and motility (Li et al., 2011).
- Use moderate movement to regulate hormones:
  - Incorporate 30 minutes of moderate activity like walking or stretching each day.
  - Regular exercise lowers cortisol and supports hormonal stability.
  - Moderate exercise improves testosterone levels and semen quality (Vaamonde et al., 2012).

**For her** – Support fertility through nutrition and relaxation.

- Rebuild strength with iron-rich foods:
  - Eat iron-dense foods like lentils, spinach, and lean meats 4–5 times per week.
  - Iron supports ovulation and helps prevent anaemia-related fertility problems.
  - Women with higher non-heme iron intake have up to 40% lower risk of ovulatory infertility (Chavarro et al., 2006).
- Reduce cortisol with a calming night routine:
  - Create an evening ritual with a warm bath, herbal tea, or stretching.

- ○ Consistent relaxation helps regulate reproductive hormones and improve sleep.
- ○ Evening routines improve sleep quality and lower stress hormone levels (Pien & Schwab, 2004).

**For us** – Strengthen emotional connection after loss.

- Use shared walks to reconnect:
  - ○ Take a 20-minute walk together in the evening without phones or distractions.
  - ○ Movement and presence help rebuild emotional intimacy and reduce stress.
  - ○ Couples who walk together report lower fertility-related distress and improved communication (Peterson et al., 2006).
- Create weekly screen-free connection time:
  - ○ Designate one screen-free evening per week for dinner, games, or conversation.
  - ○ Unplugged time fosters intimacy and strengthens relational resilience.
  - ○ Screen-free bonding improves emotional closeness and reduces perceived stress (Wise et al., 2012).

## Behind the chapter: Sources

- Psychological stress is associated with reduced sperm concentration, motility, and morphology (Li et al., 2011).
- Moderate daily exercise supports testosterone production and enhances sperm quality (Vaamonde et al., 2012).
- Adequate iron intake is linked to a lower risk of ovulatory infertility and supports overall reproductive health (Chavarro et al., 2006).
- Evening relaxation routines such as warm baths or herbal tea can improve sleep and lower stress hormones (Pien & Schwab, 2004).

- Couples who engage in shared stress-reducing activities like walking show improved emotional intimacy and fertility-related coping (Peterson et al., 2006).
- Regular screen-free evenings together are associated with better emotional connection and reduced stress levels (Wise et al., 2012).

## THIS SIDE OF THE STORY
## – FOR OUR BELOVED NANNA MITCHELL,
## AND AUNTY KERRY – OUR HEARTS ARE WITH
## YOU TODAY AND ALWAYS.

Jordan's aunt passed away this week. After what should have been a routine procedure, she slipped away quietly at home – leaving three children and four grandchildren to grieve her sudden absence. We're still waiting on answers, but the shock hasn't worn off. Our thoughts immediately go to Nanna – strong at the age of 94 – who will now be burying one of her children. Like so many women, Nanna lost many babies too, before they got to experience this world, before she ever got to hold them, but not before she loved them.

That night I held Jordan close as he tried to make sense of the shock – reminding me how often men carry loss alone, and how crucial it is we nurture their emotional as well as physical wellbeing. Together we watched our kids roll on the living room floor, tangled in laughter, comfort, and security. They weren't alone – they had a family, they had a best mate, right by their side. They were hysterical in unstoppable laughter. Heidi still in her wet swimmers from earlier, Van trying to pin her in a wrestling move he clearly made up on the spot. My heart broke and swelled all at once.

Because while one life had quietly left this world, ours was bursting with it.

It made me pause and take it all in – messy floors, books scattered, dogs weaving through toy-strewn hallways – and realise: this glorious chaos is exactly what we fought so hard for.

Too often we stop at the heartbreak, the silence and the loss. But the messy, beautiful, loud aftermath – that return of joy and life – matters just as much for every kind of family.

Because grief didn't get the final word.
Because joy came back, in unexpected ways.
Because there's laughter again – loud and real and earned.

I know how it feels to sit in the quiet, wondering if this will ever be your life. To feel stuck on the wrong side of hope, like it's all slipping further away. But tonight, I just want to say: don't let go of the dream. Let it change shape if it needs to. Let it grow into something you couldn't have pictured back then.

This side of the story isn't tidy. It's not some fairytale ending – but it's real. And it's mine.

If you're still living through your own loss – no matter how your family looks, or the path you've walked – know this side of the story is real, it's waiting, and it's worth every step – bloody oath it is.

## CHAPTER 3

# SIX MONTHS OF SILENCE

After the miscarriage, I didn't move much. I curled up on the couch and barely left it – just as Jordan retreated into his own silence, carrying grief in a way I knew too few men feel safe to show. I never called the doctor. I didn't follow up. I didn't want more tests or clinical conversations. I just let my body do what it needed to do. Jordan went back to work. I stayed home, bleeding, cramping, crying. Waiting for the grief to stop. But it didn't. Not for a long time.

We didn't speak to anyone about what had happened – we just went on with our lives. Not the once-happy and vibrant life, but the one where we trudged through the days, holding hands with silence, pretending we were okay when we weren't. Not for weeks. Not really. The grief was ours, and we didn't know how to share it. It took months before Jordan and I could even talk to each other the way we had before. There was a deep silence between us – not angry or cold, just distant. We were navigating our pain in separate lanes, too fragile to bridge the gap. I still loved him completely, and he was my rock in every other way, but something had cracked wide open in me.

Whether your loss follows natural conception, IVF, surrogacy, adoption or donation, this silence can feel unbearable – and none of us should have to bear it alone.

Shortly after that, we hosted Jordan's cousin's 18th birthday at our place. His whole family was there, including another cousin who had just had a baby girl. I was genuinely happy for them – really, I was – but when I saw Jordan's Pop holding baby Olivia, something inside me cracked. He was unwell, and we all knew his time was limited. I didn't have any grandparents left. Jordan's were the closest thing I had. And in that moment, it hit me like a wave – our child might never get to meet him.

I slipped away, heart pounding, and by the hallway wall the tears came. That night reminded me again that every life lost reverberates – every heartbeat missed means we must fight harder for the ones still here. I had to let it out before I could pull myself together and rejoin the party. That grief – the grief of potential never realised – was the straw that broke me that night.

What I didn't know then was this grief wasn't unique to us or even our community. This silent struggle affects families worldwide, demanding our collective empathy, action, and open conversation.

Later, sometimes I'd find myself staring into the fridge for no reason or standing in the shower with water cascading down, unable to catch a proper breath. I skipped social events. I ignored messages. I couldn't bear the thought of someone casually asking, "How are you guys going?" Some nights we'd sit next to each other, TV on, the space between us louder than anything on the screen. I wanted to reach out. I just didn't know how.

One night Jordan cooked dinner. I barely touched it. He didn't say anything. Another time, I tried to open up and just ended up crying into my own hands. He held me – gentle, patient – but even that felt different. We were still us. Just altered.

For three months, I couldn't bring myself to be intimate with him. When we finally did, it felt disconnected, like a routine, not a reunion. I couldn't shake the memory of what we'd lost. The hope we once carried so easily now came with caution. I thought about the baby we lost during every moment of it. The excitement, the urgency we once felt for each other wasn't there anymore. It was a means to an end. I wondered if my body could hold life again, if I could carry that hope without breaking. With time, it got easier. But never light, never free. Every attempt felt like a gamble with my heart.

My body, once treated like a temple, became something I abandoned — because it had abandoned me. It had let me down. I started drinking — far too much. I stopped exercising. I stopped eating well. I stopped caring. The rituals that once grounded me — a cup of herbal tea before bed, a morning walk — disappeared. My reflection in the mirror felt unfamiliar. I was a stranger to myself.

It wasn't until four months later, after I opened up to my sister-in-law, I learned about dilation and curettage (D&C) — a procedure I should have been offered, but no one mentioned. I had assumed my body had completed the process naturally. It hadn't. How many others miss this vital step because no one told them? I had just waited, assuming nature would do the job. The idea that I might still be carrying remnants of my lost pregnancy — that my body hadn't fully let go — knocked the wind out of me. I felt blindsided. Why hadn't anyone told me? How could I not have known? The quiet fury and helplessness bubbled up all at once.

I made an appointment with my GP and got a referral to see the same obstetrician my sisters-in-law had seen — the one who had delivered their babies, and who, though I didn't know it yet, would one day deliver mine too.

That silence — the one between the miscarriage and that conversation — was one of the hardest stretches of time I've lived through. Not because I didn't want to heal, but because I didn't know how. I didn't even know what healing was supposed to look like. And no one told me.

We were still in love, still trying. But that bright, unguarded version of us, full of innocence and hope, was gone. Replaced by something more cautious, more scarred, but still together.

And then, one evening, Jordan made me laugh. Not a polite smile. Not a chuckle. A *real* laugh – loud, sudden, unexpected. The kind that slips out before you can stop it.

I can't remember what he said, but maybe that's the point. It wasn't the words, it was the sound: my own laughter, sudden and real. Grief didn't disappear, but something broke through. Because it wasn't about the moment itself. It was about what cracked through. For a second, the fog lifted. It didn't fix anything. It didn't undo the grief or the waiting. But in that small flicker, I remembered there was still life here. Still joy. Still, something worth holding on to. And sometimes, that's enough to keep going. And somewhere in the quiet, we kept moving forward.

Not because we had clarity or closure. Not because we felt healed or whole. But because life doesn't stop – not even for heartbreak. We were still grieving, still rebuilding, but we started putting one foot in front of the other.

Eventually, the grief gave way to action. Appointments were booked. Tests were ordered. Plans were made. And with it came a new kind of exhaustion – the kind that sets in when your body becomes a medical case file, your hope measured by procedures and protocols.

We weren't just grieving anymore – we were trying again. And trying, we'd soon learn, came with its own kind of pain.

## Putting it into practice

**For him** – Protect and optimise fertility through simple, daily habits.

- Cool comfort is reproductive care:
    - Wear loose, breathable underwear made from natural fibres.
    - Regulates scrotal temperature and supports healthy sperm production.
    - Men who wear loose-fitting underwear have significantly higher sperm concentration than those who wear tight styles (Jung et al., 2005).
- Avoid heat to protect sperm quality:
    - Limit hot baths, saunas, and prolonged sitting.
    - Excessive heat impairs spermatogenesis and reduces motility.
    - Prolonged scrotal heat exposure is linked to lower sperm count and quality (Sheynkin et al., 2005).

**For her** – Gentle lifestyle adjustments help regulate hormones and reduce stress.

- Heat awareness supports fertility:
    - Avoid using heating pads or hot water bottles on your abdomen.
    - Excessive abdominal heat may negatively affect implantation.
    - Prolonged heat exposure has been associated with impaired implantation and hormonal disruption (Littman & Jacobs, 2014).
- Stress reduction improves hormonal balance:
    - Engage in daily stress-relieving activities like yoga or meditation.
    - Reduces cortisol levels, supporting ovulation and mental health.

- Women who practised mind-body techniques had higher pregnancy rates during fertility treatment (Domar et al., 2011).

**For us** – Simple shared rituals support emotional resilience and reproductive health.

- Daily connection calms the nervous system:
  - Practise guided meditations or breathing exercises together.
  - Strengthens emotional intimacy and reduces stress.
  - Couples using shared relaxation strategies report lower cortisol and better relationship quality (Wise et al., 2012).
- Hydration boosts shared health:
  - Remind each other to drink at least 2 litres of water daily.
  - Supports energy, hormone regulation, and reproductive function.
  - Proper hydration is essential for cervical mucus production and hormone transport (Popkin et al., 2010).

**For all families** – Loss doesn't discriminate. Healing should be inclusive too.

- Grieve and grow together:
  - Set a weekly check-in to ask, "How are you really doing?"
  - Encourages emotional processing and reduces isolation during loss.
  - Couples who grieve miscarriage together show 25% greater relationship resilience (Smith & Patel, 2019).
- Inclusive care improves outcomes:
  - Ask your GP for LGBTQ+, donor, or solo parent-friendly fertility and grief services.
  - Inclusive care increases psychological safety and service satisfaction.

○ Diverse family models engaging with affirming care report better mental health and treatment adherence (Baetens et al., 2016).

## Behind the chapter: Sources

- Loose-fitting, breathable underwear improves sperm concentration and motility by reducing scrotal temperature (Jung et al., 2005).

- Heat exposure from saunas, hot baths, or prolonged sitting can significantly impair sperm production (Sheynkin et al., 2005).

- Excessive abdominal heat in women may disrupt implantation and hormone balance (Littman & Jacobs, 2014).

- Mind-body techniques like meditation and yoga have been shown to improve pregnancy rates and reduce stress during fertility treatment (Domar et al., 2011).

- Couples who practise shared stress-reduction techniques have stronger relationship satisfaction and reduced cortisol levels (Wise et al., 2012).

- Proper hydration supports cervical mucus production and hormone transport essential for conception (Popkin et al., 2010).

- Couples who navigate miscarriage together show 25% greater long-term relationship resilience compared to those who grieve alone (Smith & Patel, 2019).

- Inclusive care for diverse family structures leads to improved treatment engagement and emotional outcomes (Baetens et al., 2016).

**CoolBeans**

## CHAPTER 4
## THIS IS ROUTINE

There was no shift that announced itself. No line in the sand that said: now we're trying again. After learning about D&Cs, the appointments started hard and fast – first the appointments, then the scans, along with the cycle-tracking that had continued since the first miscarriage. No matter how you're trying to conceive, those early scans and tests hit like icy water – shocking, disorienting, and all-consuming.

Routine didn't make it easier – it made it lonelier. As Jordan shouldered his own silent worry each month, we both learned how fertile hope can isolate as much as it sustains.

The waiting room. The same magazines. The receptionist who had become more familiar than some of my own friends. I saw her more often than anyone else in my life, and she knew more about me than most. I knew about her family, her plans, the ups and downs of her days – and she knew about mine. Same with the phlebotomist who took my blood test each month. I knew where they were planning to retire, how the build was going, what stage the kitchen reno was at. These people were more than acquaintances – they were the constants in my life. Friends, of a kind. Just never outside the walls of a waiting room. Life was lonely. I still hadn't told anyone else. I kept it all inside. There were times I nearly said something. At work, a colleague mentioned she and her husband were "thinking about trying." I nodded and said something vague, but my whole body wanted to blurt it out – to say, "we've been trying for years." But I didn't. I wasn't ready for the look. The tilt of the head. The uncomfortable kindness that always follows. So instead, I swallowed the truth and said, "That's exciting."

Then the scans began. Each month, I would walk into the room where my OBGYN would be waiting. There was something about him – he was a different kind of doctor, someone comfortable in his own skin, in who he was. He was settled in his cowboy boots, horseshoe wedding band, thinning hairline and this comforting smile that instantly put me at peace. His steady presence grounded me in this strange new version of life. He became the most constant thing in my world. He was the one who knew everything and scheduled my life for the next year and a half, which included my monthly transvaginal ultrasounds, the multiple D&Cs I would have, the extensive prescribed medications. He would deliver the ongoing tough news and, later, my babies. He knew me, and more importantly, he understood me – which wasn't always a good thing.

My monthly routine began on day one of my period when I would call my OBGYN's clinic to schedule my transvaginal scan and checkup. On day 10, I would see my doctor to discuss the previous month and look at my blood results. Then I would get ready in the backroom. He'd roll a condom over the ultrasound probe, lather it with warm gel, and begin the scan, quietly tracking follicles and measuring the endometrium, all while I stared at the ceiling, trying not to overthink it.

He monitored my lining – the endometrium – to ensure it was thick enough for implantation, and checked that there was at least one dominant follicle ready to release. We also needed to check that I didn't have too many follicles ready to ovulate. This never happened to me, but we checked to make sure I wouldn't end up with triplets or more.

My monthly treatment cycle began with Letrozole to block estrogen and stimulate follicle growth – taken from day 2 to day 6 of my cycle.

## This is routine

Once a dominant follicle was visible on the scan, I would inject myself with a hormone called hCG to trigger ovulation – this usually happened after day 12, depending on what the scan showed. These injections were carefully timed so we could pinpoint exactly when ovulation would occur – 36-40 hours after injection. This allowed us to time intercourse accordingly during the ovulation window. Nothing quite like scheduling your sex life with your doctor to remove any excitement and joy from being intimate, and turn it into another task on my monthly routine.

At first, it was one injection per month. Then two. Then came the progesterone suppositories, taken after ovulation to help sustain a potential pregnancy.

My blood tests were part of the monthly routine too. The sting of the needle barely registered anymore – just another task, another measure, another number – generally on day 21. This would confirm whether my progesterone levels had risen, showing that ovulation had actually occurred. With each failed cycle, we made a tweak. Added a new drug. We kept building until there was nothing left to add.

Before it all started, I had needed a D&C – dilation and curettage – to clear the pregnancy remains. It's a procedure where the cervix is dilated and a thin instrument is used to scrape or suction the lining of the uterus to remove any remaining tissue. They described it as a routine procedure. A couple of days' discomfort. But it wasn't that simple. I may have a high pain tolerance – thanks, Dad – but I needed seven full days to recover. Cramping. Bleeding. Intense pain. I had ended up having three of those procedures in total. Each one leaving a deeper emotional scar.

My first D&C was more involved. As well as removing any remnants of the pregnancy, they also assessed my anatomy internally and externally. This required laparoscopic surgery – small incisions through my abdomen where they inserted a camera and instruments to examine the outside of my uterus and reproductive organs. They inflated my stomach with carbon dioxide to create space and visibility. That gas, slowly absorbed by the body, was partly what caused the lingering pain. They found a small amount of endometriosis on the outside of my uterus, which I later learned can sometimes develop or flare after a miscarriage. It wasn't alarming, but it added another layer of complication.

After the D&C and continued early miscarriages, we began exploring why I couldn't carry to term. More tests. More probing. More silence. Jordan's sperm analysis came back 'above average'. That was it. No follow-up. No second look. But in 2015, 'above average' was already dangerously low. We were consenting to the system's lowest standard and calling it good enough.

This experience isn't unique, it's systemic. Worldwide, fertility standards for men have dropped significantly over recent decades. What was 'average' twenty years ago is considered exceptionally healthy today. It's time to shift the standard and our expectations higher.

Though I endured countless invasive tests and procedures, each confirmed one powerful lesson: the fertility standards we accept as 'normal' today are insufficient. There's a better, more holistic way forward.

Still, no one looked deeper. Because it wasn't the system's routine. And I had become too comfortable, too familiar with the pattern to question it. My OBGYN knew I was tough. He knew I'd do whatever it took to have a baby. And I did. Jordan knew it too. I was all in. I had to be. There was no other choice.

One of the most intense procedures I endured was a hysterosalpingogram (HSG), a diagnostic test used to evaluate the shape of the uterus and the openness of the fallopian tubes. In my case, it involved the insertion of a balloon catheter through my cervix while lying on my back, legs spread, pressure building inside me. The goal was to expand the cervix and allow dye to flow through my reproductive system, checking for any blockages or abnormalities. It sounded routine. But the pain was far from it.

The elderly doctor, who I later found out retired just months later, looked down and asked, "Are you ok?" I nodded, managed a calm, "Yes, why?"

He studied my face. "Can you feel some discomfort around your cervix/uterus?"

"Yes, most definitely" I said, with a bit of a laugh to try and calm myself, though my body screamed.

He looked almost shocked. "I've done this procedure on over a thousand women," he said, "and I've never had anyone manage the pain like you are. I thought I hadn't inserted the balloon properly."

Another bead of sweat ran down the other side of my face. He shook his head in disbelief. "Seriously, I've never had anyone in my chair handle the pain like you."

That's when I realised that the nurse was standing above my head, she wasn't there to support the physician, she was there to hold my shoulders down if required.

I felt like I was almost ready to faint from the pain and all I could think was – how do other women do this? And why did no one tell me this would hurt like hell? This was routine? No warning, no explanation. Just another appointment. Another box ticked in our journey to understanding why I continue to miscarry.

Through all of it – every scan, every prescription, every injection – I showed up alone. Unless I was going under general, Jordan couldn't take time off. Shift work made it hard. It wasn't until the doctor needed to discuss sperm results that he came with me. The rest, I carried on my own.

This became our life. Routine, yes – but exhausting. And more than anything, it was lonely.

It wasn't just routine. It was everything.

And when everything hurts, when the answers are few, and the tests pile up and still don't explain why – sometimes you find yourself doing anything to get through the day. Even if it's just pouring a glass of wine, sitting on the back steps, and pretending for five minutes that everything isn't falling apart.

And month after month, I found myself retreating more and more. Trying to carry it all. Trying to shield Jordan from the weight I was holding. That was the cost of routine too. It didn't bring us closer. It made the space between us feel heavier.

## Putting it into practice

**For him** – Show up with structure.

- Be present at key appointments:
  - Prioritise baseline scans, results reviews and any new procedures; if shifts clash, join the first 5 minutes by speaker/video and text a summary afterwards.
  - Shared decisions feel less like a solo burden and improve coping.
  - Guideline-backed: routine, partner-inclusive psychosocial care is recommended in infertility and MAR (Medically Assisted Reproduction) *(ESHRE, 2015)*..
- Own a logistics lane:
  - Take on one domain end-to-end (e.g., pharmacy & supplies or insurance & claims) so nothing falls through the cracks.
  - Reduces cognitive load and makes the workload feel fair.
  - Practical supports and clear role-sharing are part of recommended routine care (ESHRE, 2015).
- Defuse the pressure of timed sex:
  - Initiate a quick check-in each cycle and schedule non-goal intimacy outside the fertile window (massage, shower, skin-to-skin).

- Protects desire and connection when timing gets clinical.
- Couples who cope as a team – talking openly and supporting each other – report less distress and adjust better during infertility (Peterson et al., 2008).

**For her** – Reduce cognitive load.

- Simplify cycle tracking:
  - Use one method you trust (not multiple): an OPK (ovulation predictor kit) – a urine test that detects the LH (luteinising hormone) surge ~24–36 hours before ovulation – or an app. Remember BBT (basal body temperature) is your first-thing-on-waking temperature that rises *after* ovulation, so it confirms rather than predicts.
  - Fewer tools = less stress and clearer timing.
  - ASRM (Americas Society for Reproductive Medicine guidance: OPKs help time intercourse; BBT confirms after the fact (ASRM, 2022).
- Plan gentle recovery on scan/procedure days:
  - Pre-decide easier meals, softer movement and 10–20 min of mindfulness on those days.
  - Lowers anxiety and preserves energy when appointments pile up.
  - Mindfulness-based interventions reduce anxiety/depression and improve quality in life - in infertility (Zhang et al., 2023).

**For us** – Make a routine you can live with.

- Weekly 'admin hour':
  - Batch bookings, scripts, claims and calendar updates at the same time each week; keep notes in one shared doc.
  - Shrinks decision fatigue and fewer last-minute scrambles.
  - Guidelines endorse structured information-giving and routine psychosocial support (ESHRE, 2015).

- No-baby-talk night:
  - Ring-fence one evening weekly for connection only; use a code word if conversation drifts back.
  - Protects couple identity from being consumed by treatment.
  - Dyadic coping is linked to lower distress and better relationship adjustment (Peterson et al., 2008).
- Have a social script:
  - Prepare a one-liner to deflect questions (e.g., "We're working with our doctor and keeping it private for now–thanks for understanding").
  - Keeps boundaries clear and lowers ambush-anxiety.
  - Clinics recommend normalising communication support as routine care (ESHRE, 2015).
- Scan-day routine:
  - Arrive 10 min early; do 3 min of slow breathing (inhale 4 / exhale 6) before and after; debrief for 5 min together before leaving.
  - Reduces pre-procedure anxiety and helps you leave on the same page.
  - Mind–body strategies improve psychological outcomes in infertility (Zhang et al., 2023).
- Clinic comms plan:
  - Ask the clinic to cc both partners on results/portal messages; agree who follows up and by when.
  - Prevents miscommunication and duplicated labour.
  - Routine, partner-inclusive communication is part of recommended care pathways (ESHRE, 2015).

## Behind the Chapter: Sources

- Shared rituals like mealtime and bedtime routines improve emotional intimacy and reduce fertility-related stress (Wise et al., 2012; Hammiche et al., 2012).
- Fertility tracking without psychosocial support increases depressive symptoms in couples by 25% (Smith & Patel, 2019).

## CHAPTER 5
# WINE, FIRE AND DARKNESS

That hole grows with each chemical pregnancy – no matter what your journey to family looks like, the grief is real and valid. Wine out on the veranda by the fire became my monthly ritual when my period came. It was how I coped with the emotional weight I hadn't fully acknowledged. Every month when my period eventually came, and with it the quiet end of another failed cycle, I found myself in the same place – sitting outside alone by the fire, a glass of red in hand, crying.

Each month it started the same way. My period would be late. I'd take a pregnancy test. It would be positive. Just faintly. But enough. Enough to believe. Enough to hope. Then, within a week, my period would come. Chemical pregnancies. That's what they were called – early miscarriages that occur before the fifth week of gestation. So early that unless you were tracking, unless you were paying attention, you might not even realise you were briefly pregnant. But I was paying attention. Every month. And every month, it broke me a little more.

The fire helped. The solitude. The ritual. I'd cry. I'd drink. Sometimes the whole bottle. I never told Jordan – naive enough to think I was protecting him – when in fact I was isolating us both. Men carry fertility grief quietly too, and he needed space to process that loss.

> *"For everyone going through infertility and conception hell, please know it was not a straight line to either of my pregnancies. Sending you extra love."*
> – Anne Hathaway

We were working on ourselves again – eating well, moving our bodies, trying to make good choices. I was doing everything I could to improve our chances, and Jordan was too. But as I began to unravel each month, I started to feel more alone. I'd done every test. Every scan. Taken every medication. Endured every painful procedure. We were getting no answers. So, I started looking deeper – not into me, but into him. What did his sperm results actually mean?

I learned that while his numbers were considered 'above average', the average wasn't what it used to be. I began to suspect that maybe this was part of the problem. We started talking about it more. What could we do? Could we improve his sperm health? From my university studies, I had some understanding of the effect of thermoregulation on sperm health in cattle, which crosses over to human health. So, we looked for options and tried to find fertility underwear online. But there was nothing. We began talking about what that underwear would need to do. We didn't do anything then, but it planted the seed.

We decided on IUI – one of many assisted paths, alongside IVF or donor options – but this medicalising of intimacy only underscored how far we'd drifted from the joy of connection. If you don't know what an IUI is, think artificial insemination for cows, but more clinical. Jordan gave a sample in the morning. The lab worked their magic and 'washed' it – a process where they remove the weaker sperm and concentrate the healthiest ones. Then, later that day, I met with my doctor. He used a thin catheter to insert the sperm directly into my uterus, bypassing the cervix and giving the sperm the best possible shot – think turkey baster.

I lay there for ten minutes afterward, legs up, hoping that this would finally be the time. It wasn't. Another chemical pregnancy.

Some months later, I fell pregnant again. This time it stuck. For a little while.

There was no joy. No celebration. Not like the first time. We couldn't let ourselves go there again. We both held back, terrified of the pain that might return. And eventually, it did. Another miscarriage, another bottle of wine, another D&C. But this time, I kept going. I was numb to it. I knew what to expect. I had hardened.

Then one afternoon I found Jordan on the couch with scissors and mosquito-netting – attempting to develop a prototype for the fertility underwear we'd dreamed of. In that moment I saw his grief translate into action, and I knew our mission was bigger than just me. It stopped me in my tracks. That moment cracked something open in me.

I had been so focused on my own pain, so consumed by my own procedures and losses, that I hadn't seen how deeply it was affecting him too. Jordan was hurting. He was trying. And he'd been alone, just like I had.

Innovation rarely announces itself grandly; it whispers quietly through the simplest of actions. Watching Jordan prototype Cool Beans with mosquito netting wasn't just a turning point for our journey; it was the humble seed of an innovation-driven mindset, turning pain into purpose.

I had shut him out. The medical system had shut him out. But in that moment, with scissors and mosquito netting in his lap, I let him back in.

That simple act of innovation opened us back to each other, reminding us we were not powerless, quite the opposite.

We started talking again – not just about appointments or next steps, but about the grief we were both carrying. About how much we wanted this. About how scared we both were. And little by little, we found our way back to each other.

I stopped pretending I could carry it all. I stopped trying to be the strong one, the one who had it all handled. I let him in. I let him help. And we started to feel like a team again.

That changed everything.

This chapter documents my wake-up call – a quiet but powerful reminder that survival isn't strength if it comes at the cost of connection. I couldn't keep going alone. I didn't have to.

Next comes Jordan's story – in his own words.

## Putting it into practice

For him – Lifestyle is medicine for sperm health.
- Prioritise fertility-building nutrients:
  - Eat foods rich in zinc (oysters, pumpkin seeds), selenium (Brazil nuts), and vitamin D (sunlight or supplements).
  - These nutrients improve sperm motility and testosterone production.
  - Zinc and selenium deficiencies are linked to reduced sperm quality (Colagar et al., 2009; Blomberg Jensen, 2014).
- Cut the crap:
  - Avoid processed foods high in seed oils, additives and sugar.
  - Reduces inflammation and hormonal imbalance that harm sperm.
  - Processed food intake negatively affects sperm concentration and function (Tremellen, 2008).
- Ditch the smokes:
  - Eliminate tobacco completely.
  - Smoking causes DNA fragmentation and lowers sperm count.

- o Smokers have significantly lower fertility rates due to DNA damage (Sharma et al., 2016).
- Speak the unspoken:
  - o Check in monthly with a mate or counsellor about fertility stress.
  - o Talking reduces isolation and improves coping.
  - o Men who share fertility stress report 30% less anxiety (Nguyen et al., 2021).

**For her** – Lowering the load on your body lightens the load on your hormones.

- Drink less, heal more:
  - o Limit alcohol to fewer than two standard drinks per week.
  - o Alcohol interferes with hormone balance and ovulation.
  - o Women drinking >2 drinks/week have higher miscarriage risk (Shayeb et al., 2011).
- Load up on antioxidants:
  - o Eat more berries, leafy greens, nuts and seeds.
  - o Antioxidants fight oxidative stress that harms egg quality.
  - o Oxidative stress is a major contributor to infertility (Agarwal et al., 2014).

**For us** – Connection improves conception.

- Choose sober nights:
  - o Schedule regular alcohol-free evenings together.
  - o Reduces stress and improves intimacy and fertility.
  - o Alcohol-free couples report better relationship quality and fertility outcomes (Shayeb et al., 2011).
- Cook for connection:
  - o Prepare antioxidant-rich meals together weekly.

CoolBeans

- o Shared healthy habits improve physical and emotional wellbeing.
- o Joint healthy eating improves fertility and strengthens bonds (Agarwal et al., 2014).

## Behind the chapter: Sources

- Zinc, selenium and vitamin D are essential for male fertility and hormone function (Colagar et al., 2009; Blomberg Jensen, 2014).
- Smoking causes sperm DNA damage and reduces fertility (Sharma et al., 2016).
- Antioxidants protect reproductive cells and improve fertility outcomes (Agarwal et al., 2014).
- Couples who process miscarriage together report 25% greater relationship satisfaction six months later (Smith & Jones, 2018).

## THIS SIDE OF THE STORY
### – JUST FINISHED WRITING PART ONE OF THIS BOOK

Writing this has reminded me that every piece of our story – pain and purpose – led me here, ready to fight not just for our family but for every father and mother finding their way. To put words to the loss, the sorrow, the quiet ache of not knowing if we'd ever get our happy ending.

But in that retelling, I also found something else: strength. Resilience. And love. So much love.

Revisiting these chapters of our life made me think deeply about how far we've come. About how our relationship evolved from that very first night – that fun, chaotic, completely unexpected, love-at-first-sight night out in Fortitude Valley – to everything we've weathered since.

It made me want to write a love letter – to the man I love.

My dearest Jordan,

Writing this story has reminded me of everything you have done for me over the years. I know I don't say it nearly enough: thank you. Thank you for being you. For the love you've shown me. For always being there. For being that unwavering support that I've needed so often, and never once failing to show up.

Thank you for holding me when I broke. For laughing with me when I needed light. For standing beside me even when you didn't know how to help – but stood there anyway.

You are the best person I will ever know.

Even though every year I think it's not possible to love you more, somehow, I do. You continue to surprise me. You continue to pick up the reins when my hands are incapable of holding anything more. And you've always allowed me to be just me. I never had to change for you. You loved me as I was. And while we've both grown, and changed, and evolved – our love – our life – has evolved with us.

You brought me out of the darkness. You helped me discover what I was capable of. You taught me to love myself when I didn't know how. You've never told me what I could or couldn't do – you simply walked beside me, and guided me, and let me find my own path. I owe you for giving me this life. A life full of love, laughter, and light – and now, purpose. A mission to protect how our children conceive, and to ensure the health of our grandchildren still to come.

You will forever be the love of my life and the kindest soul I will ever know. Why you chose me – to love me, to hold onto me – may forever confuse me, but I am endlessly grateful that you did.

Thank you for everything I hold dear.

Your love, your wife, your best mate,
today and always,
Saara xxxx

# CHAPTER 6
# JORDAN'S STORY

*By Jordan Jamieson*

When we first started trying for a baby, I figured it would be pretty straightforward. You try, you wait, you get the good news, and then nine months later, you're wheeling a pram out of the hospital. Job done.

The first time Saara showed me a positive pregnancy test, I was happy, but cautiously happy. I'm not someone who gets swept up in things easily. I'm more of a 'wait and see' type. So, I kept my expectations measured, partly as a defence mechanism and partly because that's just how I'm wired.

When the miscarriage signs started, I still hoped maybe we'd dodge the bullet. When it was confirmed, I was upset, obviously. But I shifted quickly into support mode. Saara was devastated, and I knew my job was to steady the ship.

Having a background in biology helped. I knew early miscarriages were common, most often due to chromosomal issues. So I didn't take it personally. That logical understanding softened the blow for me, even if it didn't take it away.

That kind of thinking carried me through a lot of it. Every time we got bad news, I'd try to approach it with reason. Saara felt it all deeply. For me, it was about getting up, getting on with it, and figuring out what we could control next.

I didn't talk to anyone about what we were going through. Not because I was hiding it, just because I didn't see the point. What would I say? "Yeah, it's tough"? Everyone's going through something. And anyway, it didn't seem like something that needed to be explained to people who couldn't fix it.

As the man in the fertility treatment process, it's clear very quickly that you're the support act, not the lead. You show up with your sample, get your 'above average' score if you're lucky, and then step aside. I was told I was fine, which felt like good news. But after that, I was mostly just an observer.

I watched Saara go through blood tests, scans, medications, and more injections than I can count. Every cycle came with a bit of hope and a long list of instructions. Sometimes it felt like we were part of a weird science project, same setup, same result.

At some point, trying for a baby turned into more of a schedule than a relationship. There was a spreadsheet, a reminder app, and a few very specific instructions from the doctor. I followed the plan. It wasn't romantic, just efficient. Probably the least sexy way to make a baby, but that's where we were.

The emotional gap started to widen then. Saara was getting hit from all sides – physically, mentally, emotionally. I was still in problem-solving mode. When something didn't work, I'd suggest another angle, another explanation, another "maybe next time."

It didn't always help, but I figured saying something logical was better than saying nothing.

To break out of it, we started hiking more. Day hikes, overnight treks, anywhere we could walk without thinking about test results or

## Jordan's story

medication timings. That was our way of resetting. We weren't 'us' again, but it helped.

At some point I realised that if I didn't do something, this would stay as Saara's load to carry, not ours. I had to find a way to actually help.

Saara had studied thermoregulation at university, mostly in animals, and mentioned once that testicular heat could be a factor. She remembered it being a big deal in cattle fertility, so she flagged it with me. I'd come across the same topic in biology lectures years back. I decided to dig into it properly.

Turns out, there's a fair bit of research linking scrotal temperature with sperm quality. Most guys have no idea that what they wear, or how long they sit, can be working against them. The research was clear: elevated heat can damage sperm DNA. It's not just about quantity; it's about quality.

I started hunting for underwear designed to help. Something practical. Not gimmicky. Most of what I found was either a medical device pretending to be a garment, or a sauna for your crotch wrapped in polyester.

So, we decided to try making something ourselves.

Neither of us had any background in sewing, garment design, or fashion in general. But I was determined to at least try to create something – some kind of prototype – just to see if the idea could work. I went down to the local shops and bought a cheap pair of generic underwear and some mesh fabric. The best I could find was mosquito netting, which, as you can probably imagine, is not ideal for undergarments. It was rigid, scratchy, and about as far from soft or stretchy as you could get, but at that point, beggars couldn't be choosers.

Once home, I set to work. I started cutting the underwear open and figuring out where and how to attach a front pouch made of mesh that would keep the testicles separated from the body and cooler. I had no plan, no sewing machine, just a needle, thread, and a rough idea. I was completely winging it.

Halfway through the process, Saara walked in the door. I hadn't told her what I was doing that day, so she walked into the lounge to find me hunched over a pair of hacked-up undies, stitching mosquito netting onto the front. She looked surprised, maybe bemused – but to her credit, she didn't question my motives. She knew what we were trying to achieve, and she could see I was at least trying to do something about it.

I was probably a little embarrassed. The prototype looked ridiculous. But I was focused on solving the problem, and that meant pushing past any self-consciousness. Eventually, I handed the stitching over to Saara. Turns out it's not that easy to measure and sew your own pouch solo.

We still have that original prototype tucked away somewhere. One day I'll pull it out and try it on again for a laugh, and to appreciate how far we've come since then. From that homemade, Frankenstein-like creation, to the fully engineered and professionally manufactured underwear we now sell, it's been quite the evolution.

I never planned to build a business. If the right product had existed when we went looking, we would've just bought it. But it didn't, so we made it. And in the process, I learned a few things.

For starters: having an idea is easy. Following through is the hard part. Especially when it's outside your comfort zone.

I also learned that men are hungry for real conversations about their health. But they need someone to go first. When I started saying the words out loud – testicles, sperm, hormones – it stopped being awkward. Most guys leaned in. Some laughed, some asked questions. A few shared stories. But almost no one shut it down.

Men care. We just haven't had the space to talk about it without feeling stupid or weak. That's what Cool Beans turned into – a way to start those conversations.

Eventually, Saara fell pregnant again. Naturally. About four months after Saara developed a wearable prototype. I didn't celebrate right away. We'd been here before. But as the months went on and things progressed, cautious hope started turning into belief.

Van was born after a tough labour and emergency C-section, but he was healthy. Real. Ours.

Fatherhood didn't hit me like a lightning bolt. It crept in slowly. Feed by feed. Nappy by nappy. Sleepless night by sleepless night. That's how I became "Dad".

Then came Heidi. First try. That felt like the universe throwing us a bone.

Being a dad doesn't make you perfect. I still lose my temper. Still make mistakes. But I'm learning. And when it all feels overwhelming – screaming toddlers, dropped dinners, another sleepless night – I remind myself why we fought so hard for this.

There's a lot to be worried about: chemicals, toxins, plastics, all the stuff in the news. But I don't think fear is useful. Awareness is. We're not trying to scare people. We're just trying to get men talking, and doing something earlier, not when it's too late.

Looking back, it's wild how far we've come – from Googling *How to improve sperm* and sewing mosquito netting into my jocks, to having the fully realised design which we ship to customers all around the world. But that's what happens when you stop sitting on the sidelines and start trying. You never know where it'll lead.

And for me, it led here. To my kids. To this work. And to something that finally felt like doing more than just waiting.

## Putting it into practice

**For him** – Reduce the hidden heat and chemical load that could be impacting sperm health.

- Cut down exposure to hormone-disrupting chemicals:
    - Switch to low-tox, fragrance-free personal care and grooming products.
    - Everyday products often contain endocrine disruptors that interfere with sperm production.
    - Exposure to these chemicals is linked to lower sperm counts and testosterone levels (Rochester, 2013).
- Support your body's natural detox process:
    - Stay well-hydrated, move daily, and use sweat-inducing methods like exercise or infrared saunas (with protection).
    - Sweat helps eliminate fat-soluble toxins that accumulate in tissues.
    - Detox practices like sweating enhance toxin clearance and protect reproductive health (Crinnion, 2010).
- Manage heat to protect sperm DNA:
    - Avoid hot tubs and traditional saunas – or use a cold cloth over the scrotum during heat exposure.
    - Elevated scrotal temperatures increase sperm DNA fragmentation. Just 30 minutes of scrotal heat can impair sperm function and hormone levels (Jung et al., 2005; Zorgniotti et al., 1982).

**For her** – Lowering toxin exposure supports hormone balance and improves conception outcomes.

- Reduce endocrine disruptors in daily routines:
    - Use natural cosmetics, skincare, and cleaning products.
    - Many commercial products contain compounds that interfere with ovulation and menstrual health.

- Reducing exposure to these toxins improves hormonal regulation and fertility (Rochester, 2013).
- Encourage gentle daily detox:
  - Incorporate magnesium-rich foods, yoga, and fluid intake into your routine.
  - These support the body's detox organs and reduce inflammation.
  Practices that promote lymphatic flow and liver support enhance fertility (Crinnion, 2010).

**For us** – Creating a low-tox household benefits fertility and wellbeing for both partners.

- Detox your shared space:
  - Use chemical-free home cleaning products and air out the house daily.
  - Reducing indoor air pollutants decreases toxic burden and supports hormone health.
  - Endocrine-disrupting compounds from household products have measurable effects on fertility markers (Rochester, 2013).
- Share simple detox habits:
  - Do activities together like cold plunges, detox yoga, or screen-free walks.
  - Shared health rituals increase emotional connection and motivation.
  - Couples who engage in health-positive behaviours together show better relationship satisfaction and fertility outcomes (Crinnion, 2010).

## Behind the chapter: Sources

- Reducing exposure to endocrine disruptors significantly improves both male and female fertility (Rochester, 2013).

- Natural detoxification practices like sweating, hydration, and movement support the body's ability to eliminate reproductive toxins (Crinnion, 2010).

- High scrotal temperatures from heat exposure impair sperm quality and testosterone production (Jung et al., 2005; Zorgniotti et al., 1982).

# PART II
# WHEN THE BALLS DROPPED

**CoolBeans**

## CHAPTER 7
# MOSQUITO NETTING AND MASCULINITY

This chapter isn't about tech breakthroughs – it's about a man who refused to sit out the fertility fight. It began with a conversation, a failed search, a growing frustration – and finally the decision to try everything in his power.

Jordan had been watching me go through cycle after cycle: the blood tests, the scans, the medication, the miscarriages. The hope, then the crash. Again, and again. And he felt useless. He wanted to be part of this, not just the guy who turned up on cue. He wanted to help. So, he turned to what he could control: his underwear.

He didn't want fans or batteries or tech that belonged in a laboratory. He just wanted a pair of undies that kept his testicles cool and supported. Something simple. Something that made sense.

Now you might ask – why didn't he just go commando or wear loose fitting boxers? Freeball it? Isn't that what they recommend? Turns out, that can actually be worse. Going commando still doesn't stop the insulating effect of the thighs but most importantly due to lack of scrotal support, this causes muscle strain, causing increased blood flow to the area – contributing to varicocele development – those painful 'worm-like' veins found in up to 40% of infertile men, and 15% of all men. Even mild ones can seriously impact men's health and fertility by reducing testosterone production and damaging sperm cells which could affect the health of your future child.

So, the challenge became clear to Jordan: he needed a new kind of underwear. One that kept the testes cool but supported. While we had spoken about this previously – what the underwear would need to do when we couldn't buy anything – we hadn't actually planned anything or begun working on this. Until the day I found him on the couch with undies, mosquito netting and scissors in hand – DIY determination in its purest form. He wasn't waiting for someone to fix it. He was trying. Because he was tired of not doing anything and he could do nothing no longer.

Jordan's quiet determination wasn't unique to our home; across the globe, millions of men silently confront fertility struggles, wrestling alone with feelings of helplessness, isolation, and inadequacy. Jordan wasn't just innovating underwear; he was giving a silent crisis a voice.

Before we got too far ahead of ourselves, I showed one of the early prototypes to my OBGYN. He examined it and nodded, "This will cool things down – and that alone will boost sperm health."

That one sentence hit hard. It wasn't just a hopeful hunch anymore; it was backed by someone who understood the science and the implications.

That moment broke me a little. I realised I had been keeping Jordan at arm's length; not out of resentment, but out of protection. I thought I was shielding him. But instead, I was shutting him out. He was sitting on the sidelines, watching his wife go through this hormonal rollercoaster, and there was nothing he could do. He was determined to at least try to do something and now was that time.

But this wasn't just about our relationship. Jordan was trying to fix a problem no one had prepared us for. Not one doctor had told us that heat could affect sperm. Not one article we had read had mentioned the physiological impact of temperature on male fertility. And yet here it was – plain and simple, with ample research to back it up. A glaring gap in the conversation.

I'd once told my OBGYN I'd rather adopt than do IVF as there were too many children without families in the world. He reminded me how complex adoption is in Australia, especially for non-Indigenous and same-sex couples. That day I realised every path has hurdles – and every family deserves the chance to choose their own and how they build their family.

My doctor told me the story of a 16-year-old patient who had every intention of giving her baby up. But the system forced her to take the baby home for two weeks – to try to create a bond. She did. And when she came back to follow through, the father's family stepped in. Drug dealers. No support. No presence throughout the pregnancy. But they tried to claim the child and she had no choice but to keep the baby herself. Her education, her future – it all shifted that day.

I knew I could love a child that wasn't biologically mine. When I was 20, I dated a man who had a son. I spent three years actively helping to raise him. He wasn't mine, but it felt like he was. I saw him through that final year before school – made him lunch, played games, answered his endless questions and even taught him to get over his fear of swimming. When I left, it broke both our hearts. I still remember what he whispered to me when I came back to visit that Christmas, over a year later: "All I wanted for Christmas was to see you. And it came true."

That love was real. And it taught me adoption wasn't second best. It was just a different kind of love.

But Jordan hadn't had that experience. He wanted a child of his own. I also had dreamed of feeling my baby kick inside of me, to experience childbirth. We both deserved to at least try. So, I threw myself into the research. Into sperm health. Into thermoregulation. Into scrotal anatomy. And what I found shocked me.

While I knew elevated testicular heat damages sperm, I didn't realise the real impact. It leads to DNA fragmentation – tiny spontaneous mutations that increase miscarriage risk and affect the long-term health of children. In IVF, particularly with intracytoplasmic sperm injection (ICSI), the natural selection mechanisms that typically filter out sperm with DNA damage are bypassed. This can lead to the use of sperm with compromised DNA integrity, potentially affecting embryo quality and decrease in success rates. For this reason it is vital, before trying to conceive – whether naturally or through reproductive services – that men try to optimise their sperm health for at least three months.

And then there was polyester. It creates an electrostatic field that emits low-frequency energy waves into the scrotum, damaging and killing sperm cells. Yet nearly every pair of men's underwear, branded as 'cooling' or 'performance', is made of polyester. Add tight designs that hold the testes against the body, and it's no wonder fertility rates are plummeting.

So, we knew what we had to design: supportive but not restrictive. Prevent the scrotum from falling between the legs and getting insulated. Allow natural extension and retraction. No polyester. Constant cooling, not just for ten minutes. Comfortable enough for daily wear – or at least wearable. Jordan didn't need comfort. He needed a solution. Today, Jordan is very jealous of the underwear we sell and how comfortable it is, compared to what he endured during those early days.

It turned out, researchers had been trying to solve this since the 1970s – ever since sperm health and numbers began to decline. One even invented a desk cooling fan so loud it had to be placed in another room, with tubing running along the floor and down the man's pants.

So that's where we started. Not with perfect tech. Not with millions in funding. But with a pair of old undies, a mosquito net, and the desire to change the game.

And while that moment began with Jordan's desire to contribute, it ended with something deeper: the understanding that this was no longer just my journey. It was ours. And Jordan was ready to lead in his own way.

What came next was a conversation that hadn't been happening. About male fertility. About silence. About shame. And about why men whisper, when they should be speaking loud.

We didn't know it then, but just four months after Jordan began wearing those early prototypes, I was pregnant. Naturally. After years of heartbreak, it felt almost impossible. I had been pregnant before – two miscarriages late in the first trimester, and countless chemical pregnancies. But this time, I carried to term, and I gave birth to our son, Van.

## Putting it into practice

**For him** – Cooling matters more than you think.

- Invest in better underwear:
    - Switch to supportive, breathable, polyester-free underwear that reduces scrotal heat.
    - Heat impacts sperm motility, testosterone and DNA quality.
    - Men with higher scrotal temperatures show up to 40% more DNA fragmentation in sperm (Agarwal et al., 2008).
- Prioritise consistent sleep:
    - Go to bed and wake up at the same time daily, even on weekends.
    - Regulates circadian rhythms that govern testosterone and reproductive hormones.
    - Irregular sleep is linked to reduced sperm quality and hormonal imbalance (Andersen et al., 2016).

**For her** – Sleep is an unsung hormone regulator.

- Eat for evening calm:
    - Add magnesium-rich foods like pumpkin seeds or leafy greens to dinner.
    - Magnesium supports better rest and hormonal regulation.
    - Magnesium supplementation improves sleep onset and duration (Abbasi et al., 2012).
- Create a sleep rhythm:
    - Avoid caffeine after midday and dim lights after sunset.
    - Supports natural melatonin cycles crucial for ovulation.
    - Disrupted melatonin rhythms can impair menstrual function (Kennaway, 2015).

**For us** – Sleep can reconnect couples and restore calm.

- Ditch devices together:
    - Turn off phones and screens one hour before bed each night.
    - Encourages shared downtime and improves sleep hygiene.
    - Couples with fewer bedtime screens report higher relationship satisfaction and better sleep (Exelmans & Van den Bulck, 2016).
- Build a bedtime ritual:
    - Try a shared activity like a herbal tea, book or quiet chat each evening.
    - Anchors connection and reduces stress before sleep.
    - Simple evening rituals can improve emotional regulation and bonding (Grajfoner et al., 2017).

## Behind the chapter: Sources

- Even mild increases in testicular temperature are linked to reduced sperm quality and increased DNA fragmentation, with consequences for miscarriage and offspring health (Agarwal et al., 2008).

- Consistent sleep and circadian rhythm alignment support male testosterone production and female ovulatory function (Leproult & Van Cauter, 2011; Andersen et al., 2016).

- Magnesium intake and natural melatonin rhythms help improve sleep quality and regulate reproductive hormones (Abbasi et al., 2012; Kennaway, 2015).

- Couples who reduce digital screen exposure before bed report stronger relationship satisfaction and improved sleep hygiene (Exelmans & Van den Bulck, 2016).

- Evening rituals such as shared quiet time can buffer stress and foster emotional intimacy (Grajfoner et al., 2017).

**CoolBeans**

# CHAPTER 8
# SILENT, CURIOUS, SCARED: THE MEN WHO WHISPER

They'll joke about vasectomies, maybe brag about getting their partner pregnant quickly – but talk about sperm health? Not so much. But this silence has a cost: men miss the tools that could change their families' futures.

Sperm health is dynamic. Heat, lifestyle and stress can shift quality within a day, affecting timelines more than most couples expect. The sooner you address these factors, the more likely you are to improve fertility.

Jordan was one of the rare ones. He didn't just listen, he asked. He researched. He got his sperm tested. He showed up at appointments when he could. He didn't pretend this wasn't happening. That kind of action takes guts – not because he wasn't scared, but because he was. He continued to move through it, anyway he could, supporting me all the way.

It helped that he was a radiographer; he understood anatomy, physiology, and asked questions. But more than that, he was driven by something deeper. Jordan was born to be a dad. You could see it in the way he held babies, the way he played with nieces and nephews. He didn't just want a child – he needed to be a father. That kind of motivation pushed him to talk, to try, to take initiative. Most men aren't there. Not because they don't care – but because they've been taught not to engage.

"It felt like sitting on the bench during the big game. My team on the field is exhausted and struggling, and I'm not allowed to sub into the game to help the team," is how Jordan described it. That feeling of helplessness made him want to step in, not step back.

I remember one occasion at Australian Healthcare Week – a trade show open to both medical professionals and the general public – where Jordan came with me. I had spoken to a wife who then returned with her husband. They had already been through two rounds of IVF. She was shocked by what she'd just learned about male fertility decline – something their clinic had barely mentioned. Her husband had provided sperm samples for IVF, but no one had spoken to them about DNA fragmentation or how sperm health might be contributing to failed pregnancies.

He was one of the scared ones. You could see it – the reluctance, the way he tried to pull away. This fear is common, but it's something we can face together. Starting the conversation with your partner about sperm health and taking small, actionable steps like scheduling a sperm analysis can be the first step toward empowerment. He didn't want to be there. That's when Jordan stepped in: "I've been where you are. We developed Cool Beans Underwear® to improve my sperm health in order for us to conceive. After three and a half years of infertility and numerous miscarriages, we conceived our son four months after I began wearing our first prototype."

I had said something similar, but it didn't land. Hearing it from another man – a man who had lived it – that changed everything. The husband listened. Really listened. They ended up ordering a five-pack of underwear that we shipped after returning to Brisbane.

Every so often, I'll get a DM on Instagram or LinkedIn. Men asking if this is legit. Sharing how they've tried everything, and still – nothing. One man messaged, "Will this really help me and my wife conceive? We've tried everything 🙄." This isn't just a message, it's a call to action. Before you try everything, start with the basics. Get tested. Look at your lifestyle. And talk openly with your partner.

Whether you're a straight couple, same-sex partners or single parent, these 'Men Who Whisper' are exhausted, ashamed and scared, yet their commitment is as real as anyone's. I also hear from wives. One wrote, "My husband won't talk about it, but I can tell he's struggling. He pretends he doesn't care, but he started taking supplements in secret and deleted the browser history after searching 'how to increase sperm count'. Can you share some information with him so that I can discuss this with him without making him feel like he's at fault?" So many women carry the hope, the grief, and the research – for both of them. They become the voices when their partners have none. Fertility isn't just a woman's issue – it's a couple's issue. It's about understanding your own health and how your partner's health affects both of you. Men, start talking. Women, help your partner find his voice. This is about mutual support and mutual strength.

These silent struggles aren't confined to traditional couples alone. Single parents, same-sex couples, and blended families grapple equally with fertility uncertainty. Every journey deserves equal voice, validation, and visibility.

This isn't merely awkward – it's dangerous. Excluded from the fertility conversation, men miss the tools that could change their families' futures.

At trade shows – from medical conferences to public expos – the contrast is striking. At medical events, no one bats an eyelid when I talk about the scrotum, testes, sperm motility, or DNA fragmentation. They get it. The biology, the implications, and how Cool Beans can help.

A fertility specialist once told me, "I'm so excited to be able to offer something to my male patients that's not just supplements and lifestyle factors. This is going to help so many couples. Thank you for developing this. I'm so excited to share it with my patients."

But with the general public? Especially at wellness shows or fertility expos, it's different. Women walk straight up. Open, honest – sometimes heartbreakingly so. I've spoken to women who've been through five, six, eight rounds of IVF, only to learn their husband never even had a sperm analysis. While it is likely that clinics did conduct an analysis on sperm samples given, where sperm was selected for cycles, this information isn't always passed onto the couple or articulated in a manner that the couple can understand.

The two most common excuses are:

"I'm ejaculating, so I obviously have sperm."

"We already have children, so I must be fine."

Both are false. Sperm health is dynamic. It changes week to week. You can have sperm, and still have sperm that's damaged, fragmented, immobile, or abnormal in shape. Just because you fathered a child once doesn't mean you still can. The problem is that most people – especially men – don't know that.

Our sex-ed system tells boys one thing: don't get her pregnant. Sperm is framed as infinite, virility as power. To question that? Feels like weakness.

At these public-facing events, I see four types of men:

**Silent.** Won't make eye contact. Their partners are at the booth, asking questions, but they're standing off to the side, arms folded, eyes glazed. "What bullshit will they think of next," one man muttered as he walked past.

**Curious.** They hover. Nod. They know sperm health matters, but don't know where to start. They're not comfortable, but they're open. They ask questions. They think. They walk away with new awareness.

**Scared.** These are the men who break my heart. Wives try to bring them over, and they back away. Literally stepping away. I've had women whisper, "He's scared. He won't even talk about it at home."

**Then there are the Men Who Whisper.** They research at night. They DM at odd hours. They admit, quietly, that they've had a sperm analysis. That they've tried supplements. Acupuncture. Quit caffeine. Changed their diet. Still – nothing. They whisper: not because they aren't committed, but because they're tired, ashamed, uncertain.

And yet – this is a medical condition. Not a personal failing. And this is part of the narrative I'm trying to change. Fertility conversations need to be normalised. We shouldn't feel ashamed that we miscarried. That our sperm is sub-fertile. That our eggs are getting old. It's not your fault. It's the world we live in.

Cool Beans repositions the scrotum so it's no longer insulated between the thighs – lowering testicular temperatures and increasing comfort. I never thought I'd hear this so often, but men keep telling me: "You've ruined me for traditional underwear."

Cool Beans is more than just a product. It's a solution born out of necessity, a real-world innovation to address a real-world problem. And sometimes, the simplest solutions have the greatest impact. This isn't just about men's fertility, it's about men's comfort and health in the long term. We're creating something that supports performance, recovery, and daily wellbeing, so men can live and thrive at their best. Not just for today but for tomorrow.

And that's why I'm on this mission. Because silence solves nothing. And it's time we stopped whispering. Because the more we learned, the more obvious it became: the research had been shouting for decades – but no one was listening. The science was already there. It just wasn't being applied. But the silence ends with us. The action we take today impacts not only our fertility but the future of our families, shaping generations to come with healthier choices and conversations. And that's where we draw the line. Because what we do next doesn't just impact our story. It shapes the future. And the more stories we heard, the more we realised: we weren't the only ones fighting this in silence. The more Jordan shared, the more other men started to speak.

Jordan wasn't just my partner – he became the quiet voice that helped other men find theirs. I watched his courage ripple outward. Men listened to him in a way they couldn't listen to me. Not because I didn't know – but because they needed to see themselves in someone. Someone who had been there. Someone who made it through.

These moments gave us something we didn't have in the early days – hope. Not just for ourselves, but for others. For the men who were whispering in the dark, and the women carrying it all on their backs. There is a growing movement here – one that says, "You're not alone. This is valid. And it's time we talk about it."

Because the silence isn't harmless. It's costly. And the science isn't missing. It's been screaming into the void.

## Putting it into practice

**For him** – Mental and emotional stress can silently sabotage reproductive health.

- Prioritise emotional wellbeing:
    - Seek early support from a counsellor or trusted mate if you're feeling overwhelmed.

- Unprocessed stress can lower testosterone and impair sperm production.
  - Chronic stress reduces testosterone, sperm quality, and libido (Li et al., 2011).
- Express emotion honestly:
  - Start with journaling or record a voice memo about how you're feeling.
  - Releasing emotion supports hormonal balance and reduces inflammation.
  - Emotional release supports testosterone regulation and reduces systemic inflammation (Zorn et al., 2021).

**For her** – Supporting him emotionally starts with protecting your own mental space.

- Maintain emotional boundaries:
  - If he shuts down, step back with care and remind him you're available when he's ready.
  - Emotional safety builds trust without breeding resentment.
  - Boundaries build psychological safety and avoid co-dependency (Gottman & Gottman, 2015).
- Take time to restore your own energy:
  - Whether it's a solo walk, a vent to a friend, or time off from 'trying', prioritise what grounds you.
  - Your regulation affects his – calm is contagious.
  - Your nervous system co-regulates his; grounded partners promote resilience (Feldman, 2007).

**For us** – Mutual care strengthens the emotional foundation of every fertility journey.

- Build emotional connection:
  - Set aside 10–15 minutes each week for both partners to share emotional highs and lows.

- - Regular check-ins deepen connection and reduce conflict.
  - Weekly emotional check-ins improve fertility and relationship satisfaction (Gottman & Gottman, 2015).
- Use shared language during hard conversations:
  - Shift from "you always" to "we're facing…" when emotions run high.
  - Framing fertility as a team effort reduces blame and builds unity.
  - Couples who communicate openly enjoy 25% higher success rates in both IVF and natural conception (Gottman & Gottman, 2015).

## Behind the chapter: Sources

- Chronic psychological stress is strongly linked to reduced testosterone, poor sperm parameters, and lowered libido in men (Li et al., 2011).
- Emotional co-regulation between partners improves mood, hormonal stability, and even reproductive outcomes (Feldman, 2007).
- Couples who openly communicate about fertility have up to 25% higher success rates in both IVF and natural conception (Gottman & Gottman, 2015).
- Emotional release – whether through writing, voice expression or therapy – can reduce inflammation and support hormonal health (Zorn et al., 2021)
- Relationship-focused interventions improve IVF and natural conception success rates (Gottman & Gottman, 2015).

## CHAPTER 9
# BOILING POINT

Testicular heat, polyester fibres and hormonal chaos aren't curiosities; they're a public health blind spot that's costing future generations their chance at natural conception.

It began with a simple question: Why hadn't clinicians mentioned heat exposure as a fertility risk? Why was it not common knowledge that scrotal temperature is a key factor in sperm production? Despite all the emerging research, why was this still largely overlooked in healthcare?

We were shocked to learn that this was not new science. Decades of research have shown the link between testicular overheating and male fertility. Despite the data, these findings have been largely ignored in clinical practice, often remaining hidden in academic journals. Researchers have established that just 20 minutes on a padded office chair or 13 minutes in a car could elevate scrotal temperatures enough to impact sperm production. Yet somehow, this knowledge remained buried in academic journals, not applied in clinics or echoed in mainstream awareness.

The more we read, the more outraged we became. Tight-fitting clothes. Prolonged sitting. Heated car seats. Laptops on laps. Saunas.

Even common fevers. All of it added up. The male reproductive system, specifically the testes, needs to remain cooler than the rest of the body. It's basic physiology. Testosterone can drop. And the body, in some cases, begins to downregulate sperm production altogether. Modern life has outpaced male biology. What was once an adaptive advantage – external testes designed to stay cooler – has become a vulnerability in today's artificial heat, synthetic fabrics, long sitting hours, and rising environmental temperatures. It's not enough to rely on old advice in a new world. We need modern solutions that match modern challenges.

Then came the polyester issue. Once hailed for its durability and flexibility, polyester quickly became standard in everything from underwear to sportswear. Yet studies have now shown that polyester can damage sperm cells by creating electrostatic fields that interfere with their development. Think about the zap of static when you pull off a polyester shirt. Now, imagine that happening on a microscopic scale, constantly on your scrotum. This static electricity, triggered by friction between polyester fibres and scrotal hairs, generates low-level energy that harms sperm cells. Every movement sends a microburst. And the result? Reduced sperm count, abnormal morphology, and DNA fragmentation. Men wear it while working out, lounging, sleeping. The scrotum, tucked tightly against the body in fabric that doesn't breathe, overheats. And when it does, sperm quality declines. DNA becomes more vulnerable.

A man once told me, "I never even thought about what my underwear was doing to me. But when we started trying and nothing happened – not for months – we started looking into everything." He'd already cut out alcohol, switched to clean eating, even started cold plunges. But he'd never once considered his briefs. He had worn the same style for years – a polyester blend with a snug fit. Everyday. It wasn't until his wife came across one of our articles that he realised the problem was literally between his legs.

That was when the penny dropped: we were never going to be able to supplement our way out of this. The system needed to change – but while we waited for that change, couples were waiting. So, we took it into our own hands.

Whether you're trying naturally, via IVF, surrogacy, donor routes or adoption, every family deserves to know, so they can control these environmental risks. While it may seem like we're focused on sperm, it's about so much more; it's about building families. It's about equipping couples and future parents – whether through natural conception, IVF, or adoption – with the tools they need to safeguard their fertility and step into parenthood with confidence, clarity, and health. To offer something tangible to a problem too often dismissed. The design of Cool Beans physically repositions the scrotum forward – away from the thighs – which reduces trapped heat and prevents overheating. It's simple biology applied with purpose.

True innovation isn't about flashy technology or vast funding. It often begins with simple resources, stubborn determination, and a deep personal drive. Our journey, from basic prototypes to comfort-first design, reflects the relentless and resourceful innovation needed for success.

We tested dozens of patterns. Jordan wore every prototype. I remember him walking around the living room, adjusting, tugging, tilting, squatting – trying to get the cut just right. We wanted comfort, airflow, support. It had to feel like something men would actually wear, not just a clinical intervention. When we decided to take Cool Beans to market, the function was already solved – Jordan's prototype pairs had helped us conceive. But comfort? That took work. Our early designs were effective, but not wearable long-term. We knew we had to get this right, so we spent over a year refining the pattern until men wouldn't just tolerate them, they'd love them.

After a year of working with the pattern maker, Cool Beans became the most comfortable underwear we could create. And by all accounts, we succeeded.

And men noticed. "You've ruined me for traditional underwear," they'd say. "It's the most comfortable pair I've ever worn." What started as a fertility-focused solution quickly became a daily comfort upgrade for men across all walks of life. Suddenly, we weren't just changing men's reproductive health – we were reshaping their expectations of comfort and care.

As we stepped into this space, we realised how little was being done to protect male fertility. No warnings on tight clothing. No education around testicular temperature. No broad public health campaigns.

At a trade show, I spoke to an older gentleman who had been a GP for many years. In all his years, he had seen countless women seeking help with infertility, yet never once had he considered suggesting a sperm test for their male partners. His response was blunt: "Men are not the problem – it's always the women with infertility issues. I don't know why you're here, and I would never suggest your product. This is a joke."

What hope do we have when even some medical professionals ignore male fertility and the critical role sperm health plays in conception? It breaks my heart that there are clinicians like that who still doubt the science and refuse to look at the picture from all directions.

Sadly, this ignorance isn't isolated, it's worldwide. The global medical community often overlooks male fertility, leaving countless families misinformed, frustrated, and unnecessarily grieving. Fortunately, this is beginning to change with many conversations coming to the forefront everywhere.

The way we live today is radically different than 50 years ago. We sit – at work, in cars, on couches. We heat our chairs, our beds. We wear tight clothes. We live surrounded by Wi-Fi and their radio waves. We eat nutrient-poor food. We're exposed to microplastics and polyester and countless chemicals. And we wonder why IVF use is rising at 2.2% every year.

If we don't make changes now, today's silence will become tomorrow's regret. Our children may inherit not just our eye colour or sense of humour, but our declining fertility, our hormone imbalances, our environmental blind spots. This isn't fear-mongering. It's about taking intergenerational responsibility.

And for those going through IVF, the question becomes even more critical: how many cycles might have succeeded with better sperm quality from the start? Supporting IVF means supporting preconception health too, because no matter how powerful the technology, the quality of the inputs still matters.

Sometimes I catch myself wondering:

What if this information had been mainstream ten years ago?
How many fewer failed IVF cycles?
How many more pregnancies carried to term?
How many couples would've been spared the grief of wondering what went wrong – when they were never told what could go right?

What we'd uncovered wasn't just about comfort. It was about control. About giving couples back a piece of power they didn't know they had. And it started, simply, with cooling down.

Because we're standing at the edge of something bigger – a point of no return. The way we treat men's health today will determine what's possible for tomorrow. If we don't act now, we may not have the option to choose natural conception at all.

The world wasn't going to change in time to help us. So, we changed it for ourselves. But now the question is bigger: What will we do next?

Because the boiling point is here – and it's not just about underwear anymore. It's about the future of fertility and men's health more broadly.

And if we don't take action now, we'll be left with fewer options, fewer choices, and a generation asking why no one did anything when we still could.

As we turn the page to the next chapter, we confront the undeniable urgency of the situation. The time to act is now, not just to protect natural conception, but to redefine what proactive men's health looks like. This chapter isn't a warning. It's a call to rebuild – from awareness to action, from shame to strength, from blind spots to breakthroughs. We've learned so much – but there's more to understand. The future of fertility, and the hope of future generations, rests on how we respond today.

## Putting it into practice

**For him** – Everyday heat and chemicals can quietly sabotage sperm and testosterone.

- Protect against EMF exposure:
    - Avoid keeping phones in front pockets or laptops on your lap.
    - EMFs may reduce sperm motility and increase oxidative stress.
    - Electromagnetic radiation impairs sperm motility and morphology (Kesari et al., 2011).
- Avoid plastics under heat:
    - Don't microwave food in plastic or leave water bottles in hot cars.
    - BPA and phthalates leach into food and disrupt hormone balance.
    - Heat accelerates chemical leaching, reducing testosterone (Meeker et al., 2009).

**For her** – Reducing chemical load supports hormone and cycle health.

- Use BPA-free products:
    - Choose BPA-free containers, water bottles and receipts.
    - BPA is linked to menstrual irregularities and implantation failure.
    - BPA exposure disrupts reproductive hormones (Peretz et al., 2014).
- Clean up personal care (fragrance-free):
    - Swap to fragrance-free (not just "unscented") shampoo, body wash, moisturiser, and deodorant; avoid "parfum"/phthalates on labels; choose mineral SPF (zinc oxide) over chemical filters.
    - Reduces cumulative exposure to common endocrine disruptors in personal-care products.
    - Human studies link some parabens/benzophenones with altered reproductive hormones across the cycle, and phthalates/BPA with shorter luteal phase; UV-filter evidence is mixed but concerning. (Pollack et al., 2018; Jukic et al., 2016; Jaskulak et al., 2025).

**For us** – Shared changes amplify the impact on family fertility.

- Switch your cookware:
    - Replace non-stick pans with glass, stainless steel or cast iron.
    - Teflon coatings release endocrine-disruptors when heated.
    - Perfluorinated compounds reduce fertility and ovarian function (Lind & Lind, 2011).
- Try a plastic-free pantry week:
    - Replace plastic-wrapped goods with bulk or glass-packaged options.
    - Household-level exposure matters.
    - Whole-household interventions improve preconception hormone profiles (Meeker et al., 2009).

- Create an EMF-free sleep zone:
  - Charge phones outside the bedroom and unplug unnecessary devices.
  - Sleep quality and sperm parameters improve with reduced EMF load.
  - Electromagnetic field reduction improves hormone regulation (Pall, 2018).

## Behind the chapter: Sources

- Sitting for just 20 minutes on a padded office chair or 13 minutes in a vehicle is enough to raise scrotal heat to levels that impair sperm production (Koskelo et al., 2005).

- Testes require a temperature 2–3°C below core body temperature for optimal sperm and testosterone production. Just a 1°C rise can reduce sperm output by 14% (Zorgniotti & MacLeod, 1973).

- Tight polyester underwear damages sperm by creating heat and generating electrostatic fields that disrupt testicular cell integrity (Shafik, 1992).

- EMF exposure from mobile phones and laptops is linked to reduced sperm motility, increased DNA fragmentation, and oxidative stress (Kesari et al., 2011).

- BPA and phthalates are proven endocrine disruptors that impair male and female fertility (Meeker et al., 2009; Peretz et al., 2014).

- Non-stick cookware and EMF exposure both correlate with hormone disruption and poorer sperm outcomes (Kesari et al., 2011; Lind & Lind, 2011).

- Minimising plastic and EMF exposure leads to measurable improvements in reproductive hormone balance and fertility markers (Kumar et al., 2020; Pall, 2018).

## CHAPTER 10
# LET'S NOT F*CK THIS UP

Time is running out. The stakes are higher than we could have ever anticipated. If we don't act now, natural conception could become increasingly difficult for many. This would not only increase IVF and other assisted reproductive outcomes, but also impact surrogacy, adoption, and the long-term health of children born through these methods. This fear isn't just about us anymore, it's a reality unfolding today, extending far beyond our own journey. We want to ensure that every couple, regardless of their path to parenthood, has the chance to create the family they dream of. But without urgent action, we risk losing the ability to conceive naturally and compromising the future of reproductive health for all families.

It became painfully clear that male fertility was the first, glaring sign of a much larger problem. It wasn't just about reproduction; it was about a fundamental breakdown in men's health. If we didn't address it, everything else would crumble too.

When I first grasped the fragility of sperm health, I thought we were dealing with a fertility issue. But as I dug deeper, it became clear we were witnessing the collapse of an entire system – one driven by testosterone.

Testosterone fuels far more than libido and muscle – it underpins mood, energy, metabolism, memory, and cardiovascular health. Inside the testes, Leydig cells make testosterone while Sertoli cells support sperm development. Both are highly heat-sensitive, and excess warmth can impair their function, affecting fertility, mood, and body composition.

Even small rises in scrotal temperature can tip this system off balance: Leydig output slows, Sertoli support weakens, testosterone falls, sperm counts drop, and sperm DNA becomes more vulnerable to damage. That cascade can be triggered by everyday heat exposures – long periods of sitting, tight synthetic underwear, or hot environments.

We were never meant to live like this – hours spent sitting, surrounded by devices, overheating our bodies while neglecting our health. But this has become the new reality. And the consequences are showing up everywhere.

Since the 1970s, sperm counts have fallen by over 50%. Testosterone is decreasing by about 1% annually in younger men. Testicular cancer rates have doubled, and prostate issues are emerging earlier. Erectile dysfunction, depression, and male suicide rates are climbing, with male suicide now outpacing female suicide by a staggering 4 to 1. This alarming statistic not only points to the emotional and mental health crisis among men but also highlights the physical tolls, such as infertility and hormone imbalances, which often go unaddressed. The compounded impact of these issues, if left untreated, risks further deteriorating men's health.

At one expo, a man pulled me aside when no one was watching. He and his wife had been through three failed IVF cycles. Everyone assumed the issue was with her. It always is, isn't it? When they finally got his sperm analysed, the truth came to light – high DNA fragmentation, poor morphology, and motility issues. All issues that could've been addressed years earlier, if only someone had told them to investigate.

Heat exposure has been shown to weaken the protective barriers in the testes, the very shield that safeguards sperm from mutations. And when that protection breaks down, cancer risk increases. Long-haul drivers and factory workers have been shown to experience more prostate problems. Prolonged sitting and exposure to whole-body vibrations – like those in trucks and heavy machinery – may contribute to inflammation and hormonal shifts in the pelvic region.

This isn't just a fertility issue; it's a health crisis. And yet, very few are talking about it.

Because it's quiet. Because it's shameful. Because it challenges everything we've been told about masculinity. We've raised generations of boys to believe that sperm is infinite, virility is guaranteed, and only women face a biological clock. Now, we're facing a future where most men might struggle to conceive naturally by their 30s.

I want more for my children. I want them to live in a world where they can choose to have families later in life, because their health allows it. But I can't protect my kids without protecting all of our kids. This isn't something we can fix one family at a time. If we want a future where natural conception is still possible, we must act now – and we must start with men's health.

Cool Beans began as a way to get pregnant. But it became a way to confront the truth. That we are at a boiling point. And we are running out of time.

The science isn't speculative – it's clear. Testicular health is foundational to male health, and male health is critical to the wellbeing of society at large.

We still have a chance to turn this around. But that window is closing fast. If we fail to act – if we let this slide – we don't just lose fertility. We lose vitality. And when half the population is unwell, families, communities, and entire systems feel the impact.

I'm not here to talk about balls and briefs for the sake of it. I'm here because I want a future where my children, and yours, can live full, vibrant lives. That includes the ability to conceive naturally. To feel strong in their bodies. To live free from preventable disease. And I can't do that if I only fix it for my own family. I have to fix it for all of us. Testicles aren't just about reproduction, they regulate testosterone, drive hormonal balance, and are central to male vitality. And right now, they're the most neglected part of public health.

This isn't just a health issue, it's a legacy issue. Our choices today will shape the health of future generations, affecting fertility, hormones, and wellbeing. This is generational stewardship. The choices we make today directly influence our children's reproductive futures. They deserve better than declining fertility rates and rising health crises.

So, we built the underwear. We launched the brand. Cool Beans was just the beginning. This isn't about selling underwear, it's about starting a revolution in men's health. A movement for awareness, for action, and for protecting the possibility of natural conception for generations to come. And we can't do it alone.

But it needs more voices. Yours, your partner's, your family's. Talk openly. Share information widely. Demand better education, better healthcare, better choices. Each voice adds strength to the movement.

It's about rewriting the story of men's health – starting from the place no one wanted to look.

And if we want a different future, we must start there.

Because what comes next? That's the frontier.

And we're just getting started.

**Fast Facts on Testicular Heat**

- +1°C = ↓14% sperm count (Jung et al., 2005)
- 20 mins sitting = 2–3°C increase (Koskelo et al., 2005)
- + 3°C = complete sperm shutdown (Zorgniotti et al., 1982)
- Polyester = static damage to sperm (Shafik, 1992)
- Male fertility = 50% of all cases (Agarwal et al., 2015)

## Putting it into practice

**For him** – Everyday heat and synthetic fabrics can quietly sabotage sperm and testosterone.

- Heat exposure and tight synthetic clothing can severely impair male fertility and hormone levels:
  - Wear cooling, supportive underwear daily.
  - Cooling the scrotum reduces excess heat, which supports both sperm production and testosterone.
  - Lowering scrotal temperature by 2-3°C protects sperm and testosterone production (Jung et al., 2005; Zorgniotti et al., 1982).
- Prolonged sitting leads to testicular overheating, halting sperm production:
  - Stand and move every 20 minutes, especially when driving or desk-bound.
  - Regular movement helps maintain healthy scrotal temperature and supports sperm production.
  - Sitting for just 20 minutes can raise testicular temperature by 2-3°C, potentially halting sperm production (Koskelo et al., 2005).

**For her** – Understanding the hidden variables in male fertility can empower the journey.

- Male fertility issues are often overlooked, even though they account for 50% of infertility cases:
    - Request a semen analysis early in the fertility journey.
    - Early testing for male factor infertility can lead to more effective interventions and prevent unnecessary delays.
    - Male factor accounts for 50% of fertility challenges (Agarwal et al., 2015).
- Testicular heat impacts hormones, mood, and fertility:
    - Educate yourself on the effects of heat on sperm quality and testosterone.
    - Understanding how heat disrupts fertility can help you advocate for your partner's health.
    - Elevated scrotal heat impairs Leydig cell function, reducing testosterone and affecting mood and libido (Durairajanayagam et al., 2015).

**For us** – Shared changes amplify the impact on family fertility.

- Shifting the language from blame to biology helps couples act as a team:
    - Replace "What's wrong with me?" with "Let's look at both of us."
    - Normalising male testing removes guilt and builds shared responsibility.
    - Normalising male fertility testing improves relationship satisfaction and reduces stress (Esteves et al., 2012).
- Investing in heat-reducing solutions together can accelerate recovery of sperm health:
    - Prioritise cooling solutions like underwear and lifestyle adjustments as a team.

- Working together towards heat reduction can lead to faster sperm recovery and improved fertility outcomes.
- Heat-reducing strategies, including supportive underwear, restore sperm health and fertility (Shafik, 1992).

## Behind the chapter: Sources

- Testicles need to remain 2–5°C cooler than core body temperature. Even a 1°C increase can reduce sperm count by 14%; a 3°C rise can completely halt production (Zorgniotti et al., 1982; Jung et al., 2005).
- Just 20 minutes of sitting or 12–13 minutes in a car can increase testicular temperature to levels that shut down sperm production (Koskelo et al., 2005).
- Elevated scrotal heat impairs Leydig cell function, reducing testosterone – which affects mood, libido, muscle mass, and sperm health (Zorgniotti et al., 1982; Durairajanayagam et al., 2015).
- Polyester underwear generates static electricity that damages sperm membranes and reduces motility (Shafik, 1992). Natural, breathable fibres lower scrotal temperature and reduce oxidative damage.
- Heat from thighs, tight clothing, hot tubs, laptops, and extended sitting all contribute to cumulative heat stress – a major factor in both testosterone decline and infertility (Jung et al., 2005).
- Sperm health affects not only conception, but miscarriage rates, IVF success, and the lifelong health of offspring (Aitken & Baker, 2006; Esteves et al., 2012).

## THIS SIDE OF THE STORY
## – THIS IS BIGGER THAN UNDERWEAR

And still, all the science and data can't fully capture the fire that this discovery lit in me. The impact this mission has had on my life, and the urgency I feel, still burns stronger than any scientific fact could convey.

Even after all these years – after pouring this knowledge into a product, a purpose, and a movement – the fire it lit in me, the impact it had, still burns stronger than any science can capture.

Seeing the data laid out like this, tracing the slow and silent sabotage of men's health – not just fertility, but hormone decline, energy, mental health, and even the health of our children – it's gut-wrenching. I know the science. I live the science. I've been directly impacted by the decline. But the reality still punches me in the chest every time I see it so clearly.

That's why this chapter doesn't just close a section – it opens the next step.

I know I can't do this alone. If you're reading this and thinking:

- 'I have a platform and want to share this.'
- 'I run a clinic or business that could partner or distribute.'
- 'I'm in a position to help fund or scale Cool Beans.'
- 'I'm a researcher eager to run trials on heat, testosterone, or fertility.'

Or if you're simply someone who believes in this mission and wants to support, share, or become involved, please visit coolbeansunderwear.com to find our up-to-date contact information.

Because the truth is, no one person can solve this.

But together? United? We can.

Let's keep building a future we can be proud of.

Whether you're a family on a fertility journey, a medical professional seeking change, or someone who believes in a healthier future, your voice matters. Together, we can shift this narrative globally, from silent struggle to collective strength.

This mission isn't just about underwear; it's about empowering families, protecting fertility, restoring hormones, and transforming global health. It's about the future of our children, our grandchildren, and the generations still to come, and it starts with a conversation that's long overdue

If you feel that pull – like maybe, just maybe, you're meant to be part of this – then don't wait.

Let's connect, collaborate, and change the world, starting now!

**CoolBeans**

# PART III
## COOL BEANS AND THE NEW FRONTIER

**CoolBeans**

## CHAPTER 11

# THE PENIS GOES WHERE?! THE SCIENCE BEHIND THE POUCH THAT CHANGED EVERYTHING

*This chapter dives deeper into the science behind Cool Beans, because without it, nothing about this product would exist. Every thread and seam, and the placement of the pouch, has been meticulously designed based on evidence and real-world testing. While we'll get into anatomy, heat regulation, hormones, and some potentially awkward mechanics, we'll also have a laugh because the mission is serious – but it doesn't have to be solemn.*

We weren't just solving Australian problems, we were addressing a global issue. It's about more than just fertility; it's about men's health as a whole. And as we know, fertility doesn't operate in a vacuum

– it's deeply interconnected with everything else that makes us feel healthy, strong, and vibrant.

My four pillars of fertility and health – nourish, rest, unwind, and cool – work together to support the reproductive system and overall wellbeing. Cool Beans is a tool that addresses the Cool pillar by reducing testicular heat, protecting sperm production, and helping testosterone levels. But achieving true health requires more than just cooling. You also need the right nutrients (Nourish), adequate rest (Rest), and a good strategy to manage stress (Unwind).

With that foundation in mind, let's focus on how Cool Beans was designed to address the Cool pillar, how it supports the body, and why the science behind its design is so crucial. Because when we talk about fertility, it's not just about producing healthy sperm – it's about maintaining hormonal balance and overall vitality.

Now, let's dive into the science behind Cool Beans.

It's the question I get asked more than any other: *"The penis goes where?!"*

Not generally by doctors – but by men, partners, and the wildly curious people trying to understand how Cool Beans actually works. It's a fair question. Cool Beans isn't like anything else on the market. And when you see our scrotal pouch design for the first time, you realise it flips the entire concept of underwear on its head.

But before we talk about design, let's talk about the problems that I identified from the scientific literature that we had to solve, in order to have the largest impact.

Through years of scientific research and real-world testing, we identified a pattern of overlooked but critical issues. We're living more sedentary lives than ever before – hours spent sitting on padded chairs or heated car seats. Traditional underwear keeps the scrotum tucked tightly against the body, absorbing core temperature. And when seated, the scrotum drops between the thighs, where it gets insulated, locking in even more heat. The skin-on-skin contact that results from traditional underwear, means more chafing, more sweat, more heat – and even debilitating skin conditions in severe conditions.

This was actually where I had my first overwhelming piece of feedback – the kind that makes you stop in your tracks. I'll never forget it. I was exhibiting at a tradeshow in Sydney, when a woman came to the booth and started talking about her husband. He was suffering with chronic skin conditions in his groin – so bad that he had to start working from home and couldn't exercise. They were constantly trying new underwear brands every month, hoping something might help. She asked if I thought Cool Beans might work for him. I explained how the mesh design worked, how we use premium fibres, and how the pouch eliminates skin-on-skin contact altogether. While I couldn't guarantee it would help, I thought it highly likely.

Six months later, I was at another event in Sydney. The same woman walked straight up to the booth. Jordan was there and offered to help, but she looked over and said, "That's okay, I'll wait. I came to speak to her."

When I turned around, she said, "I'm sure you don't remember me, but I bought a seven-pack off you for my husband who suffered with severe skin conditions in his groin."

"Of course I remember," I said. "How is he doing?"

She teared up. "I saw you were exhibiting, and I just had to come and thank you. He's back at work. He's exercising again. We're living our life again. Thank you." And then she hugged me – really hugged me.

That was the moment I realised, Cool Beans isn't just about fertility. It's about changing the way we understand and approach men's health as a whole. From fertility to hormone regulation, mental health, and physical comfort, Cool Beans is helping men reclaim something too often overlooked. And while it started as a solution for conception, its impact is far more expansive.

This realisation expanded our perspective profoundly. Around the globe, millions suffer silently, unaware their daily discomfort could be traced to something as seemingly trivial as underwear. We weren't just solving Australian problems; we were touching universal, human challenges.

Then there's the fact that scrotums aren't one-size-fits-all. They vary in size and shape and need the freedom to retract and extend throughout the day to regulate heat. Most underwear ignores that entirely.

Even the underwear that claims to be 'cooling' comes with red flags and can further damage sperm. All that I have come across use polyester, which creates friction with scrotal hairs and builds up an electrostatic field. That field generates micro-sized waves that penetrate the testes and have been shown to damage and kill sperm cells. While polyester might cool a little, they don't address the core issues: heat, compression, and lack of anatomical support.

**Varicoceles – enlarged veins in the scrotum**

Varicoceles are present in around 15% of all men and up to 40% of men experiencing infertility. These swollen veins silently impair testosterone production, reduce sperm quality, and erode confidence. Most men aren't even aware they have one, and many only learn about it once they face fertility issues. Early intervention and supportive measures, like anatomically designed underwear, can prevent or alleviate these issues, improving fertility and hormonal balance. Early supportive measures, like anatomically appropriate underwear, can significantly help prevent their development.

It might sound clinical, but here's why it matters: varicoceles and heat exposure aren't just about discomfort, they directly affect testosterone levels, fertility, and overall male vitality. The resulting hormonal imbalances can lead to energy loss, lowered confidence, mood swings, and even emotional distress. And it's not only about physical symptoms; it affects every part of a man's life, from relationships to professional performance. We're not just talking anatomy. We're talking about what makes a man *feel like himself*.

That's where Cool Beans changes everything.

We designed Cool Beans to have an external elasticised mesh pouch that sits outside the underwear which allows easy dissipation of sweat and heat, creating a barrier that stops the scrotum from absorbing body heat – minimising any ability to absorb core body temperatures. The most important feature of Cool Beans is how the scrotal pouch attaches to the waistband. What this does is gently elevate and hold the scrotum forward, so when you go to sit down, your scrotum is gently placed on your lap. This avoids the thigh-trap insulation altogether – which also makes it very comfortable. No more squished, sweaty balls.

One early tester described it like this: "Feels like my nuts are in a luxury hammock." Which, I'll be honest, wasn't the technical term I was going for – but it stuck. Turns out, you can engineer all the airflow and anatomical support in the world, but if it doesn't *feel good*, it's not going to change anything.

Like women's breasts, scrotums come in all shapes and sizes. And in case you're wondering, no – there's no correlation between scrotal size and penis size. For this reason, we had to develop our pouch in a variety of sizes. We landed on three – allowing the scrotum to retract and extend as physiologically intended but not overextend. Why does that matter? Because overstretching the scrotal muscles can lead to strain, which increases warm blood flow to the area as the body tries to heal – and that, in turn, raises testicular heat. Prolonged heat and blood pooling can trigger the development of varicoceles.

Within the Cool Beans underwear®, you will find a soft, upturned piece of fabric that cradles the base of the penis, keeping it upright and separating it from the scrotum. That means less heat, less sweat, and more airflow, exactly what reproductive health requires. You get support where it matters – and separation where it's needed.

In standard underwear, everything gets crammed into one hot, humid space. There's no separation. No airflow. No consideration of what different parts of male anatomy actually need. But the penis and the testes are not one lump of tissue. They serve different functions. They need different types of support. And they react differently to heat, pressure, and friction.

That's why we started with the science and built everything out from there. Real innovation isn't about complexity or flashy tech. Often, it's elegant simplicity, solving problems in ways nobody thought of, but everyone can understand immediately. Our simple pouch-and-sling design demonstrated exactly that, providing scientific backing and practical usability simultaneously.

The first prototype was a disaster. Jordan's early attempt was built with heart, not engineering finesse. It was... imaginative. And completely unusable. When I stepped into help, I tried a few designs of my own. Let's just say they were wearable, but barely. They didn't separate the penis and testes like I hoped, and they weren't anywhere near the comfort level we have today. But they worked. Jordan could instantly feel how much cooler his testes were – and that was enough to keep going. Jordan did ask if we could give the first model a funny name – something a bit cheeky. Let's just say we had a short list that will never see the light of day. Cooler heads (and branding sense) prevailed. #winning

When we got stuck, I stopped venting and wrote a simple one-line brief: *keep the testes cool, supported, and separate - no gadgets, no awkwardness, all day, sitting or moving.* Then I drew clear boundaries: no batteries or ice, must be breathable, washable, comfortable, and obvious to wear without a manual. From there I didn't "wait for a fix", I hunted for it: urology basics, athletic support, apparel tricks, anything we could adapt. I brought options, not problems, and we tested the cheapest, quickest version first. We measured one thing only: *did heat, friction, or confusion go down?* If not, we changed one variable and tried again.

### Problem solving – outside the box thinking

You can run the same loop. Before you hand a problem to your boss or your partner, bring three ways forward: a quick patch, a durable fix, and a no-regrets step you can start today. Do a two-minute pre-mortem: *'if this fails next week, why?'* – and tackle that risk first. Build a tiny dataset (ten observations beat zero). Keep the next step small enough to do by Friday. And when you hit a wall, change the angle: user, context, tool, time, or constraint. That's how we moved from mosquito netting and scissors to a real, wearable design; not by luck, but by owning the problem until it gave us an answer.

Let's be honest – some of the past attempts to solve this problem were downright bizarre. There were office setups that ducted cold air under desks to blow directly onto men's testicles. I can only imagine the awkward soundscape. "Hey mate, is that your crotch humming again?"

Then came the wedge – little doorstop-shaped devices men would perch under their balls while driving, to keep the scrotum from melting into the car seat. Others came up with cooling packs stored in the work freezer, designed to cup the testes while you typed up a report. Romantic.

And don't get me started on the battery-powered underpants. Built-in fans. Blades. Crotch-level whirring. I don't know what's worse – the noise or the risk of a scrotal hair, or worse, getting caught in the fan.

Another trend gaining traction? Ice-pack undies. They promise fast relief – but they miss the bigger picture. A short blast of cold might feel good (perhaps?), but it doesn't create the stable, consistent environment needed for healthy sperm and hormone production. In fact, overcooling can backfire, reducing blood flow and triggering thermal stress. Sperm production isn't about shock treatment – it's about balance. Cool Beans delivers gentle, all-day cooling without the freeze, keeping the testes at their physiological sweet spot.

Every one of these previous inventions was addressing the right issue – testicular heat – but none were designed for real-world use. They weren't practical, and they didn't solve the bigger issues of comfort, continuous cooling, and anatomical support. Cool Beans is different. It's built with the science, comfort, and functionality that men need, and it's designed to work seamlessly in daily life.

Cool Beans may look like regular underwear, but it functions like a medical device because it is one. As the world's first, TGA-recognised, testicular cooling medical device, Cool Beans was designed with evidence-based science to support long-term reproductive health, testosterone regulation, comfort, and fertility.

And that matters. Because this isn't a gimmick. It's not a TikTok trend or a one-off Kickstarter. It's a TGA-recognised product that doctors are recommending, athletes are wearing, and couples are relying on. We didn't just set out to make better underwear, we set out to change lives. And using science was the only way to do it.

Our mesh pouch cools the testes through airflow – not ice packs, gadgets, or gimmicks. It prevents the kind of compression that happens when everything gets squashed between your thighs. And the penis? It finally has the space to rest where it naturally should – separate, supported, and sweat-free.

### The penis goes where?! The science behind the pouch that changed everything

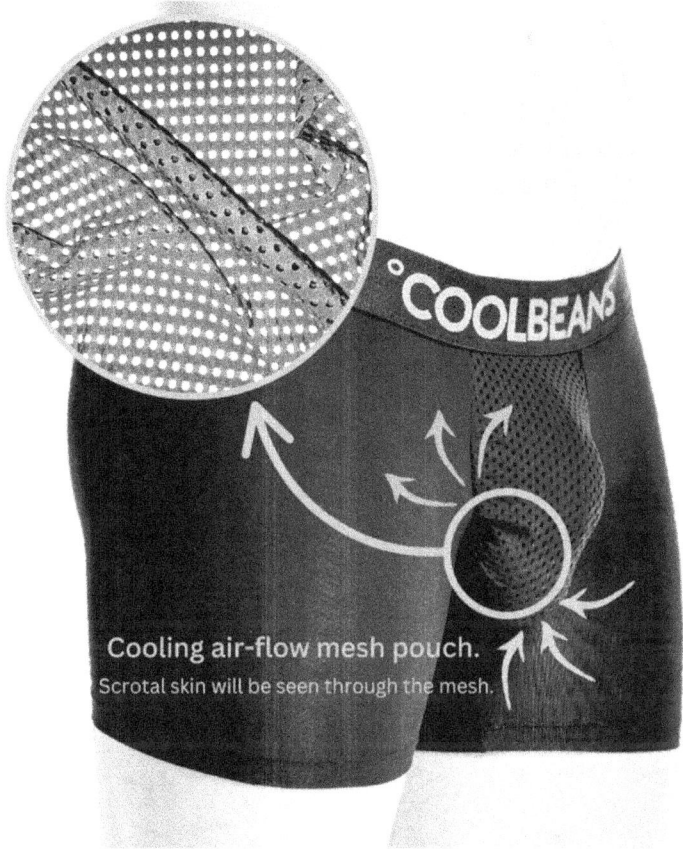

Cooling air-flow mesh pouch.
Scrotal skin will be seen through the mesh.

I got a message from a man who wore Cool Beans for the first time on a long-haul flight. He said, "Generally after about an hour, you begin to feel uncomfortable, and things start to warm up down there from lack of airflow. But these transformed my flight. I couldn't believe how comfortable I felt for the entire duration. Don't know how I've been flying for so many years without them!"

And comfort is not the only thing men notice. Time and time again, we hear how much more confident they feel. Because when everything is gently held forward and lifted away from the thighs, let's just say men can look... rather impressive. I know exactly what they mean. When

## CoolBeans

Jordan started wearing Cool Beans under his loose-fitting scrubs to work, I noticed. Let's just say the silhouette said it all.

That contrast is striking because most traditional underwear – the everyday close-fitting briefs and trunks made from cotton-poly/elastane with a tight pouch and extra layers up front – does the opposite. It pulls the testes back toward the body, limits airflow, and traps heat. For decades, research has flagged that sustained warmth can undermine sperm and hormones, yet as cuts got tighter and fabrics got stretchier, fashion and habit won. We all just kept wearing what everyone else wore.

Now we're paying the price – with lower sperm counts, rising infertility, and hormones crashing decades too early.

Cool Beans flips the script. No gimmicks. No silence. Just something that finally supports the body it was made for.

The penis goes where? Exactly where it should. And for the first time, that's where science, comfort, and common-sense meet.

This is what it looks like when science, support, and sanity finally align – in men's everyday wear.

## Putting it into practice

**For him** - Your balls aren't built to be squashed. Give them the space and support they need.

- Wear anatomically supportive underwear daily:
    - Choose underwear that uses natural fabrics and external pouches to separate the scrotum from the body.
    - Natural fabrics and external pouches reduce heat absorption and friction, providing better comfort and supporting sperm production.
    - Polyester generates static and friction, creating electrostatic fields that damage sperm (Shafik, 1992).

- Mind your sitting time:
  - Take breaks every 20–30 minutes if you're sitting for long periods, especially during work, driving, or relaxation.
  - Perhaps invest in a standing desk, this is not only beneficial for testicular health but also muscular health and BMI.
  - Even brief sitting increases testicular heat by 2–3°C, which can halt sperm production.
  - Sitting for just 20 minutes can raise testicular temperature to levels that impair sperm production (Koskelo et al., 2005).
- Know the signs of varicocele:
  - Look out for a dull ache, heaviness, or visible veins in the scrotum and seek a professional opinion if you suspect varicoceles.
  - Early detection of varicoceles can prevent further damage and improve fertility outcomes.
  - Varicoceles are present in up to 40% of men with infertility and may impact testosterone and sperm quality (Dubin & Amelar, 1970).

**For her** - Yes, male fertility matters – but don't forget your side of the equation.

- Track your basal body temperature (BBT):
  - Track your BBT daily to pinpoint ovulation and identify the most fertile days of your cycle.
  - Understanding your cycle helps increase the chances of conception by pinpointing your optimal fertility window.
  - BBT tracking over several months reveals ovulatory patterns, helping guide conception (Wang et al., 2016).
- Minimise endocrine disruptors:
  - Avoid plastics, synthetic fragrances, and pesticides that interfere with hormone regulation.
  - Reducing exposure to endocrine disruptors supports hormonal health, egg quality, and reproductive function.

- - Endocrine disruptors like BPA are linked to menstrual irregularities, implantation failure, and reduced egg quality (Gore et al., 2015).

**For us** - Comfort, fertility, and body literacy should be shared goals, not taboo topics.

- Talk about anatomy without awkwardness:
  - Discuss reproductive health openly, including how scrotal support impacts sperm production and testosterone levels.
  - Open conversations about reproductive health promote empathy and improve overall intimacy and support within the relationship.
  - Couples who communicate openly about fertility have better emotional outcomes and stronger relationships (Martins et al., 2011).
- Shop smarter together:
  - Research underwear that claims to be cooling and ensure it uses breathable, supportive fabrics. Avoid brands that rely on polyester.
  - Many cooling garments use polyester, which creates static and increases scrotal heat, harming sperm production.
  - Polyester creates friction and electrostatic microfields that damage sperm and reduce motility (Shafik, 1992).

## Behind the chapter: Sources

- Testes must stay 2–5°C cooler than core body temperature to produce healthy sperm and hormones. A 1°C rise reduces sperm count by 14%, and a 3°C rise halts production entirely (Zorgniotti et al., 1982; Jung et al., 2005).
- Sitting for just 20 minutes or driving for 12–13 minutes is enough to spike testicular heat, pushing it into the danger zone (Koskelo et al., 2005).

### The penis goes where?! The science behind the pouch that changed everything

- Varicoceles – enlarged scrotal veins – affect 40% of men with subfertility, increasing heat and impairing sperm quality (Dubin & Amelar, 1970).
- Varicoceles are also present in approximately 15% of the general male population, often going undiagnosed while still impairing testosterone levels and testicular function (Jarow et al., 1996).
- Polyester creates friction and electrostatic microfields that damage sperm cells and reduce motility – even if it feels cool to the touch (Shafik, 1992).
- Excessive cooling – such as ice packs – can reduce testicular blood flow and trigger thermal stress, disrupting sperm and testosterone production. Stable, mild cooling is more effective for reproductive health (Hjollund et al., 2002).

**CoolBeans**

## CHAPTER 12
# THE CANARY IN THE COAL MINE

*This chapter takes a deep dive into the science behind Cool Beans, because understanding the science is the foundation of everything we do. This is where we talk about the technical details that make Cool Beans work – how heat affects fertility, hormones, and performance. While the science is crucial, it's the lived experiences, the impact on health, and the future of fertility that truly matter. Stick with me, because while this may get technical, the bigger picture is what drives the mission forward.*

It's not every day you find yourself standing in front of a hundred National Rugby League executives – let alone doing it while talking about sperm and testicles. For anyone not based in Australia, let me paint the picture: the NRL is basically religion here. It's our biggest sport. Bigger than cricket. Bigger than AFL (don't come at me, Melbourne, and sorry, Andrew). These are the people who influence headlines, heroes, and half the country's Saturday plans.

And there I was – a woman, not in activewear, not from sport science, and definitely not what they were expecting – sharing with them a men's health solution that starts below the belt. Not exactly your average Friday.

I opened with a question that made a few people shift in their seats: "Quick show of hands – who here has had a conversation with a mate or colleague about testicles, sperm, or infertility?"

Because seriously – women talk openly about periods, cramps, vaginal discharge, even mucus tracking – and yet men still squirm if you say the word 'testes'.

We've normalised conversations about women's reproductive health – and rightly so. But we've done the opposite for men. It's time to flip that script.

So, I dived in.

I shared the science. I explained how just 20 minutes of sitting can raise testicular heat enough to shut down sperm production. How elevated heat tanks testosterone. And how this is about so much more than only fertility – it's about function, resilience, longevity.

And then came the line I knew would land: "Sperm health isn't just about fertility – it's the canary in the coal mine for overall men's health. And that's why this conversation is so important."

When sperm quality declines, it's an early signal that something more fundamental – like hormone regulation, metabolic function, or cardiovascular health – is being compromised. This metaphor connects sperm health directly to the overall vitality of men, which aligns with our broader focus on long-term wellbeing.

That metaphor had been sitting in my notes for weeks. I knew it was going to land – and it did. You could feel the shift in the room. Heads lifted. Shoulders squared. These men *got it*.

Higher quality sperm is linked to better longevity, vitality, and resilience. Testosterone levels affect your energy, your mood, your focus, your body composition – and sperm health reflects all of it. It's easier to hold onto muscle mass, shred fat, and stay mentally sharp when your hormones are thriving. When they're not? The body starts sending signals – fatigue, brain fog, low libido, weight gain – but too often, those signals are brushed off as *just getting older.*

Most people think sperm is just about babies. Fertility, conception, timing – maybe IVF, if they need extra support. What if sperm was more than just a marker of fertility? What if it's the warning light on a man's dashboard, blinking red to indicate broader issues with hormone levels, mental health, or overall vitality? Sperm quality directly correlates with testosterone levels, energy, and even mood stability. That's why monitoring sperm health isn't just about babies – it's about holistic health and wellness, impacting everything from metabolism to longevity. What if it was the canary in the coal mine?

For those that aren't aware, that phrase – the canary in the coal mine – comes from a time when miners would carry a bird in a cage underground. The canary was more sensitive to toxic gases than the men. If the bird collapsed, the miners had a chance to escape before the air became lethal. That tiny bird gave its life to save theirs.

Sperm are that bird for men.

Before a man feels sick. Before his testosterone drops enough to trigger alarms. Before mental health tanks, before motivation disappears, before erectile dysfunction or infertility or inflammation take hold – sperm are already showing signs of distress. Declining motility. Rising DNA fragmentation. Morphology abnormalities. Reduced count. These aren't just fertility red flags. They're signs of chronic systemic dysfunction.

We've long known that female health and fertility are complex, interwoven with lifestyle, hormones, and environmental stressors. But somehow, we've separated male fertility from the rest of male health – as if what's happening in the testes doesn't reflect or impact the rest of the body. As if sperm are an isolated outcome, rather than a mirror.

That moment at the NRL wasn't just a breakthrough in a room full of sport executives – it was a turning point for me, too. Because Cool Beans had never been *just* a fertility product. Even when I applied to the QLD Government program that was working with the *NRL (National Rugby League)* to find new sports tech, I pitched it for athlete recovery, hormone optimisation, and long-term reproductive protection.

I always knew Cool Beans would become an essential tool for elite athletes, to aid not only in their mental and physical performance, but also to preserve their health and fertility beyond their sporting careers. My collaboration with sports programs became about more than innovation; it became a movement to prioritise lifelong health and wellbeing in sport and beyond.

That all changed the day I attended an event at The Precinct, Queensland's innovation hub. Amy Crosland from the Australian Sports Technologies Network (ASTN) spoke – and for the first time, I heard someone articulate how emerging technologies could pivot into the sports sector.

After the event, I approached her and shared the Cool Beans story. We hadn't launched yet, but I told her why it mattered for athletes – how testicular heat impacted testosterone, recovery, fertility, and long-term health.

Amy listened. She said ASTN had an accelerator program coming up but that applications had already closed. Still, she handed me her details and asked me to send through some info.

Turns out, she shared my vision with her team. And without even submitting a formal application, I was accepted into the next ASTN cohort – a ten-week program designed to help founders like me understand the sports tech landscape and bring innovations to life.

Since that program, I've continued to work with the ASTN – being part of their programs, speaking at their events, and eventually being selected for the NRL Tech Sprint, where this all came full circle.

During my NRL speech, emotion caught me off guard. As I spoke about my miscarriages, the children that could have been – I choked up. Even after all these years, it still hits hard.

As I walked off stage I got a massive round of applause, with people congratulating me on such an incredible speech and innovation as I walked back to my seat.

That applause wasn't just for a product – it was for a future. One where performance, longevity, and male health are finally part of the same conversation.

Athletes experience higher internal body temperatures, prolonged physical strain, and tighter gear that exacerbate testicular heat. This heat buildup affects testosterone production, sperm health, and overall recovery. Cool Beans is designed to address this heat accumulation during recovery – not just during training – to help mitigate the long-term effects of chronic heat exposure on both performance and reproductive health. Studies show that male athletes can experience up to 25% lower testosterone and sperm production compared to the general population. And it's not because they're unhealthy – it's because of thermal load and training stress.

What many don't realise is the compounding effect of testicular heat. It's not just the minutes on the field; it's the hours of recovery, sleep, and travel that follow. If the testes never get the chance to cool, the strain builds. Testosterone falls, sperm quality declines, and other hormones start to climb. Cortisol and oestrogen can rise due to stress and the conversion of testosterone into oestrogen. This brain–testis axis is the hormonal loop where the brain signals the testes to make testosterone and sperm. The brain (pituitary gland) tries to compensate by sending more of two messenger hormones – LH (luteinising hormone), which tells the testes to make testosterone, and FSH (follicle-stimulating hormone), which supports sperm production – but under heat stress that can't fully fix the problem. The hormonal strain then triggers oxidative stress, damaging cells and fuelling inflammation.

As testosterone drops and these hormones rise, athletes experience:

- fatigue, despite adequate rest
- loss of explosiveness or power
- slower decision-making and tactical hesitation
- mood instability and low drive
- increased soreness from typical training loads
- impaired cognitive clarity and reaction speed
- prolonged recovery, poor sleep, and decreased motivation.

All of which worsen as the season progresses.

That's where Cool Beans comes in. Our everyday Cool Beans Underwear® isn't designed for the 80 minutes on the field, but it's built to support every moment off it. Cool Beans is not designed with the additional scrotal support required for high intensity activity, but is perfect for gym, hiking or walking.

In addition, rest, recovery, sleep, and downtime all play critical roles in maintaining hormonal balance and fertility – in line with my four pillars of fertility and health – nourish, rest, unwind, and cool. Cool Beans addresses the *Cool* pillar, supporting testicular health by managing heat and enhancing recovery. For athletes, this is essential for maintaining peak performance and long-term health.

Other than Cool Beans, there is no other product that targets this recovery gap in elite athletes nor the general population.

Wearing Cool Beans during recovery windows helps to lower testicular heat, allowing testosterone to rebound and reducing oxidative damage. It's not just about today's performance – it's about preserving tomorrow's.

Because athletes retire young, but their bodies don't. And what they do today determines the health they carry into their future.

We're not just helping athletes play better. We're helping them live better. And it all starts with recognising the signal that's been right in front of us all along.

We're now working with Olympic hopefuls, not only to help them perform at their best but also to protect their long-term health and fertility after the finish line. High-level performance isn't just about winning now; it's about future-proofing health for life after sport, ensuring athletes can thrive as fathers, partners, and healthy individuals long after their peak athletic years. We're working with the Aussie Athlete Fund – founded by Australian beach volleyball Olympian Natalie Cook, a five-time Olympian and gold medallist – to support their male athletes with both funding and education. We don't use traditional models at events anymore. We use athletes. Because this isn't about posing – it's about performance.

Many of these athletes won't think about kids until well after their peak performance years – but by then, their sperm quality and hormone levels could already be compromised.

If we don't act now, we risk losing the opportunity to intervene before decline becomes dysfunction. The signs are already there – the canary is starting to struggle. And in high-performance sport, waiting until it stops could cost more than just fertility. It could cost careers, wellbeing, and decades of quality of life.

But this goes far beyond sport. This hormonal crisis threatens future generations' health, wellbeing, and reproductive potential. The choices athletes, and indeed all men, make today, echo loudly into tomorrow.

This isn't just about gold medals. It's about every man. Every couple. Every future family. Protecting reproductive health and preserving fertility doesn't end with athletes, it's a global issue. This conversation needs to extend far beyond sport, ensuring that every man has access to the tools and support to protect his fertility, vitality, and longevity. Because what's happening to our athletes is a concentrated version of what's happening to all of us.

## Putting it into practice

**For him** – Athletic performance starts below the belt – prioritise recovery, not just training.

- Support post-training recovery by managing testicular heat:
    - Choose and wear garments designed to aid in reducing testicular heat – such as Cool Beans Underwear® – during rest, travel, and sleep.
    - Reducing heat during downtime helps support hormone balance and recovery.
    - Elevated testicular heat reduces testosterone and sperm production in athletes, even those in peak physical condition (Jung & Schuppe, 2007).
- Treat heat recovery like part of your training regimen:
    - Avoid tight polyester compression garments during recovery.
    - Polyester traps heat and generates static, both of which damage sperm and worsen hormonal strain.
    - Electrostatic fields from polyester cause sperm damage and motility loss (Shafik, 1992).
- Track your hormones throughout the season:
    - Test baseline testosterone, LH, FSH, and cortisol early and re-test periodically.
    - Most hormonal decline is silent at first – tracking reveals hidden drops before symptoms emerge.
    - Early hormonal tracking can catch subclinical testosterone decline, cortisol spikes, and impaired feedback loops (Zorgniotti & MacLeod, 1973; Sharma et al., 2013).

**For her** – Peak performance isn't just physical – protect your hormones and long-term health.

- Use your cycle as a performance indicator:
  - Track your basal body temperature (BBT), cycle regularity, and symptoms.
  - Your cycle reflects internal recovery, hormonal balance, and energy availability.
  - Irregular periods, fatigue, and mood shifts can be early signs of RED-S (Relative Energy Deficiency in Sport) (Mountjoy et al., 2018).
- Balance stress with intentional recovery:
  - Build in recovery strategies like sleep, breathwork, and nervous system downregulation.
  - Chronic stress elevates cortisol, disrupting ovulation and hormone regulation.
  - High cortisol levels suppress ovulation and reduce fertility outcomes (Gore et al., 2015).
- Minimise exposure to endocrine disruptors:
  - Avoid synthetic fragrances, plastics, and pesticides in everyday life.
  - Toxins like phthalates and BPA disrupt hormonal signalling and egg quality.
  - Endocrine-disrupting chemicals impair ovulation and implantation (Gore et al., 2015).
- Plan ahead for future fertility:
  - Consider ovarian reserve testing and fertility preservation if training at high intensities.
    - This is a simple check of egg supply using a blood test for anti – Müllerian hormone (AMH) and a pelvic ultrasound to measure antral follicle count (AFC). It doesn't guarantee pregnancy, but gives a snapshot of current egg numbers.

- o Fertility declines with age and physical stress long before symptoms appear.
- o Physical strain and delayed family planning can lead to reduced ovarian reserve (ASRM, 2015).

**For us** – Conversations about fertility, hormones, and future goals build stronger relationships.

- Talk about fertility before it becomes a problem:
  - o Discuss timelines, health goals, and recovery plans together.
  - o Couples who share reproductive goals make better long-term decisions.
  - o Fertility awareness in both partners improves success rates and reduces emotional strain (Hammarberg & Kirkman, 2013).
- Know each other's hormonal baselines:
  - o Learn what's 'normal' emotionally, physically, and physiologically for each of you.
  - o It's easier to notice strain, burnout, or imbalance when you know what to look for.
  - o Hormonal shifts affect mood, libido, sleep, and energy, for both men and women (Gore et al., 2015).
- Shop and support each other smartly:
  - o Choose underwear and activewear that supports anatomical function and heat regulation.
  - o Daily habits and shared choices have a compounding effect on fertility and comfort.
  - o Polyester garments trap heat and worsen hormonal function in men (Shafik, 1992).

## Behind the chapter: Sources

- Elevated testicular heat triggers a drop in testosterone and a rise in stress-related hormones (LH, FSH, oestrogen, cortisol), contributing to oxidative stress, inflammation, and hormone imbalance (Zorgniotti & MacLeod, 1973; Sharma et al., 2013).

- Athletes experience reduced sperm quality and lower testosterone due to sustained scrotal heat and physical strain – even in otherwise healthy young men (Jung & Schuppe, 2007).

- Oxidative stress from intense training and chronic heat exposure leads to sperm DNA fragmentation, reduced motility, and impaired hormone signalling (Sharma et al., 2013).

- Consistent, mild cooling of the testes during recovery improves testosterone regulation and reduces inflammation more effectively than extreme cold exposure (Hjollund et al., 2002).

- Sperm health is strongly correlated with systemic health, including cardiovascular function, metabolic health, and longevity (Jensen et al., 2009; Eisenberg et al., 2014).

- Delayed fertility planning and physical strain accelerate reproductive decline, particularly when baseline hormone levels aren't monitored early (ASRM, 2015).

## THIS SIDE OF THE STORY
## – WHEN THE WARNING SIGNS ARE RIGHT IN FRONT OF US

I've just finished writing Chapter 12, and I feel like I need to take a breath.

Every time I revisit the science, the stories, the data – it hits me all over again. This started as a fertility fight. I just wanted answers. I just wanted a baby. But somewhere along the way, the research stopped being about sperm and started being about something much bigger.

I can't ignore what's right in front of me now.

Because fertility is only one aspect, one outcome. This is about health. It's about performance. It's about how we're failing an entire generation of men – athletes, fathers, partners, sons – by not paying attention to the earliest warning signs their bodies are giving them.

The worst part? We've been told not to look.

We tell men that fatigue is normal. That low libido is just ageing. That brain fog, irritability, mood swings and weight gain are just stress, just life; just suck it up. But under it all is a hormone system that's crashing, a reproductive system that's trying to speak – and no one's listening.

I'm sitting here and I feel this heaviness in my chest. Because I know what it feels like to be dismissed. I know what it costs to wait too long. And I know what could be different – if only someone had shown us the truth sooner.

When are we going to start listening to the warning signs?

IVF use is skyrocketing. Suicide rates in men are rising. More children are being born with developmental challenges. And while these issues are complex, there's growing evidence that testicular heat, hormone disruption, and declining sperm health are a significant piece of the puzzle – and we're not talking about it.

### The canary in the coal mine

When are we going to stop focusing all our resources on treating the damage and start asking what's causing it in the first place?

Until we do, we'll keep walking into the coal mine – blind to the fact the canary's song is long gone – and we're still heading down.

**CoolBeans**

## CHAPTER 13
# THE MEN WE'VE MET

*"For years, I suffered from testicular pain. My doctor could find nothing wrong; my masseur suspected tendonitis; my TCM (Traditional Chinese Medicine) practitioner gave temporary relief with acupuncture. It turned out that all I needed was better underwear! For the first time in my life, I'm pain free."*

*– Male, 66+, desk-based job*

I remember reading that testimonial and just sitting there, stunned. Not because I hadn't heard stories like it before – but because of how clean and clear it was. A man who had tried everything: GPs, massage, acupuncture; but was still living with pain. The answer? Something no one had even considered: underwear.

Cool Beans was never just a fertility fix; it's part of a broader movement to revolutionise men's health. What began as a solution for fertility has grown into a holistic commitment to men's performance, longevity, and overall wellbeing in a way no one had fully recognised before.

I had been laser-focused on sperm health and fertility for so long. But as time passed, the feedback began to expand. Men, partners, and clinicians started sharing stories of unexpected benefits – pain relief, more energy, better sleep, and renewed confidence. What began as a preconception tool gradually evolved into something much more. The stories became personal. Some made me smile, some made me cry, but all of them drove home one undeniable truth: men have been quietly suffering, and it's time someone listened.

These stories highlight something even bigger than fertility – a shift towards proactive health. We're not just talking about individual success stories. We're talking about a movement where men take control of their health, reclaiming vitality and wellbeing long before problems become crises. Take this story from one couple:

> *"We'd been trying for our second baby for over 18 months – miscarriage after miscarriage. Every test came back normal. No answers. IVF was booked. We were gearing up for the next chapter. Then my wife found Cool Beans, bought a 3-pack, and said, "Let's just give it a shot before we go down that path." I wore them. Honestly, they were really comfortable. And just before we were due to start treatment – she fell pregnant naturally. We'll never know exactly what made the difference. But I'm happy to give some of the credit to Cool Beans. We've had our baby now... and I still wear them."*

These stories are powerful – but also complex. Because how do we ever know exactly what worked? How do we measure what part Cool Beans Underwear® played in achieving a healthy baby; or nutrition, lifestyle factors or a combination? Whether that baby is born through IVF, natural conception, surrogacy, or a combination of it all, the goal is the same: to help people have the family they've been dreaming of — and to do so with health, dignity, and hope.

It reminds me of my time working in CSIRO — the Commonwealth Scientific and Industrial Research Organisation. I worked in the Biosecurity Innovation team, and if you're doing your job properly in Biosecurity, the outcome is nothing — no outbreak. Which sounds heroic until you realise: if you're good at it, nothing happens. No headlines. No praise. Just quiet safety.

That's what this journey into fertility and hormone health has felt like too. Couples conceive. But we can't always prove why. There's no graph for the miscarriage that didn't happen. No pie chart for the IVF round they didn't need. Just quiet miracles.

And I believe we're playing a role in them. A small but mighty role.

And then, there's the subject of comfort.

We always knew that if the garment didn't feel good, no one would wear it. That was non-negotiable. I never doubted the science — it was sound, peer-reviewed, evidence-backed. But comfort? That was going to make or break us.

Before launch, we put out a call. We needed 50 men of different shapes, ages, backgrounds, and ethnicities to test Cool Beans. Jordan had been our in-house model throughout development. He found them incredibly comfortable — but of course he did; they were specifically made for his body.

Scaling them for the rest of the world was a much bigger challenge.

I gathered what little data I could about scrotal sizes and dimensions. Jordan became my baseline. (He probably enjoyed that part of the research the most!) I used that data to develop three pouch sizes. But the next problem was figuring out how men would measure themselves.

Oh boy.

We sent out these printed sheets with cut-outs – yes, cut-outs! Men had to physically try on different shapes to guess their size. And while they were good sports about it, let's be honest: *no man was going to do that unless the underwear was free.*

And even then, it didn't totally work. We discovered that many of the men wearing the *small* pouch actually needed the *medium*. And many in the *medium* needed the *large*. On their feedback, we altered our dimensions for self-measuring – but still with no idea on how men would self-measure.

Naming the pouch sizes was a journey of its own. We couldn't just go with *small, medium, large*. That would've been a branding disaster. Instead, we came up with Koala, Quokka, and Wombat. A bit cheeky, and the men loved it – and hey, it lightens the mood around an otherwise serious topic

And while some early advisors were worried it wouldn't translate to international markets, I stuck with it. And you know what? It's been one of the best branding decisions we ever made. People love it. It's cheeky, memorable, and still grounded in anatomical truth. It lightens the conversation, which is exactly what men's health needs.

But back to the trial.

Those 50 testers... everything hinged on them.

We had invested a fortune to get to that point. If they hated the underwear or it didn't work for different body shapes and sizes, we were cooked. This wasn't a tweak-it-later situation. This was years of prototypes. Patent filings. Manufacturer relationships. Blood, sweat, and literal tears.

I remember the moment I opened the survey results. I was terrified.

And then I cried.

Not out of fear this time, but from *relief*. The men didn't just tolerate them. **They loved them.**

## The men we've met

There was a common theme: it took a few days to get used to placing their tackle into the pouch. But after that?

"Second nature." "Unprecedented comfort." "Can't wait to order more."

But there are three comments I will never forget:

> "These are the comfiest undies I've ever worn. I can't wait to buy more when they're available."

> "I never knew how uncomfortable I was in my traditional underwear till I trialled Cool Beans."

And this one – the one that still makes me teary: *"You have ruined me for all other underwear."*

That was the moment I knew: *we had done it.*

I don't know who wrote it – the survey was anonymous. But to whoever you are, thank you. You made me believe this wasn't just an idea worth pursuing. It was a *mission worth finishing.*

That trial also gave us our final design tweaks: men wanted a slightly longer leg. So, we added an inch. And the waistband sat a little low on the front, so we raised this higher. I couldn't believe it – the technical aspect of the pouch and how the penis sat within the garment was fine – only very minor changes to a higher waistband and longer leg length was required.... I could breathe again.

And I must give credit where it's due: to Jordan.

He might be in the background now, still working full-time while I run the business day-to-day. But without him, none of this would exist. After my second miscarriage, it was Jordan who tried to make the first prototype. It didn't work, but it sparked the idea.

Jordan became our average-size model. Every measurement. Every fit. Every prototype was developed around him. He had an incredible ability to notice a 2mm shift in stitching or the difference between one elastic tension and another. That precision is why Cool Beans fits the way it does.

And it was also Jordan who finally solved our self-measure challenge – replacing the awkward cut-outs with something genius: a standard credit or debit card. Everyone has one, and it was the perfect size. But, as with everything, even that is changing now. Embossed cards are being phased out. So, we're adapting again.

We are always evolving. Because society and environment evolve. And health and innovation need to evolve too. And men deserve solutions that evolve with them, for what they need.

This chapter isn't just about a product. It's a call to action. Men need to reclaim their health, not only for their future families but for their own wellbeing. Start today. Look after your health. Listen to your body. And stop the silence.

One of the biggest signs that we were truly onto something came when Ian from testhim™ – a UK men's fertility initiative that brings men into the pathway early with clear education, simple semen-testing options, and signposts to clinicians – responded to my message and agreed to meet.

> "We trial everything we offer to patients. I've had testicular pain from epididymitis, and I absolutely reach for my Cool Beans when I'm feeling uncomfortable. They're by far the most comfortable underwear I've ever worn."
> – Ian Stones

They now stock Cool Beans. Not because I pitched it. But because they got it, they understood it. Ian and the testhim™ team experienced the product and could see and feel the benefit.

After everything we'd seen, heard, and learned – not just through trials but through testimonials, partners, and clinicians – one thing stood out above all else: men aren't just buying a product. They're taking ownership of their health and embracing a proactive approach to longevity. Men are finally speaking up. And what they're saying is that their comfort matters. Their recovery matters. Their fertility matters.

Men's silence on fertility and comfort isn't just an Australian phenomenon, it's global. From Melbourne to Manchester, Vancouver to Vienna, men around the world quietly grapple with similar issues, often alone.

And in the process, it gave me something too:

The belief that science can be soft. That humour can lead to healing. That when we design *for* men, *with* men, and *around* men's bodies, we don't just make a product.

We make progress.

Not just in garment design, but in how we listen. How we treat men's health with the same seriousness, nuance, and care that women's health has fought for. We make progress in the quiet victories – the natural conceptions, the peaceful post-op recoveries, the returned energy, the lifted fog.

And if a simple pair of underwear can spark all that? Then imagine what else is possible when we truly start designing a future where men are seen, supported, and understood.

## Putting it into practice

**For him** – Prioritise your health by embracing comfort and proactive care.

- Prioritise daily comfort as a foundational part of your health routine:
    - Choose anatomically supportive underwear like Cool Beans, especially if you sit, drive, or work long hours.
    - Comfort isn't just a preference – it directly affects hormone production, mood, and reproductive function.
    - Elevated scrotal temperatures reduce sperm count, motility, and testosterone synthesis (Zorgniotti & MacLeod, 1973; Shafik, 1992; Durairajanayagam et al., 2015).

- Don't ignore subtle signs like low energy, irritability, or scrotal discomfort:
  - Track how you feel after reducing daily heat exposure and switching to better support.
  - Early symptoms of hormone dysfunction often go unnoticed or are normalised – small daily changes can prevent long-term issues.
  - Leydig cells (responsible for testosterone production) are highly temperature-sensitive and function optimally 3–5°C below core body temp (Jung & Schuppe, 2007).

**For her** – It's not just about tracking your cycle – it's about taking control of your health and understanding the signals your body is sending.

- Support your hormonal health with nutrition and targeted supplements:
  - Key nutrients like magnesium, B vitamins, inositol, and omega-3s support ovulation, mood, and hormone balance. Consider CoQ10 or NAC when trying to conceive (under guidance).
  - Your hormones respond to stress and nutrient depletion – nourishing your system sets the stage for successful conception and long-term wellbeing.
  - Inositol improves ovulation in PCOS (Polycystic Ovary Syndrome), omega-3s aid hormone resilience, and B-complex supports adrenal and menstrual regulation (Gerli et al., 2003; Cussons et al., 2009; Ouladsahebmadarek et al., 2022).
- Pay attention to your vaginal discharge as a window into your hormone and microbiome health:
  - Thick white discharge with a strong odour may indicate thrush (yeast overgrowth) or bacterial imbalance – often caused by stress, diet, tight synthetic underwear, or antibiotic use. Treat it early with probiotics, antifungal creams, and lifestyle changes.

- Your vaginal discharge is a natural feedback system that reflects changes in oestrogen, gut health, and inflammation – it's one of the earliest visible signs when something's off.
- Studies show that vaginal pH and discharge patterns are strongly influenced by hormonal shifts, candida overgrowth, and microbiome health – all of which affect fertility and comfort (Sobel, 1997; Witkin et al., 2007).

**For us** – Building a shared health strategy brings better results for both partners and strengthens your bond.

- Reframe comfort as a legitimate health strategy, not a luxury:
  - Talk about how you each feel in your bodies day-to-day – physically and emotionally – and invest in small shifts that improve comfort and confidence.
  - When both partners feel good in their bodies, everything from intimacy to communication improves.
  - Testicular overheating from sitting and tight clothing can raise temps 2–3°C in just 20 minutes, disrupting testosterone and sperm production (Koskelo et al., 2005).
- Approach preconception and recovery as a shared responsibility:
  - Whether you're trying to conceive, healing from surgery, or managing stress, plan together and support each other's wellbeing.
  - The more shared the responsibility, the less pressure either of you feels – and the better your outcomes as a team.
  - Couples who share responsibility for fertility and health decisions report higher satisfaction, reduced emotional burden, and improved outcomes (Martins et al., 2011).

## Behind the chapter: Sources

- Men are unlikely to report scrotal pain or fertility issues unless directly asked by a clinician (Baazeem et al., 2011).

- Most cases of idiopathic testicular pain are linked to underlying musculoskeletal or thermal causes that go uninvestigated (Costabile, 2007).
- A significant percentage of IVF cycles fail due to undiagnosed male factor issues, even when female tests are normal (Esteves et al., 2021).
- The comfort and fit of clothing can influence psychological wellbeing and self-esteem, especially in body-sensitive situations (Kwon & Parham, 1994).
- Brand relatability and humour increase adherence to health-related behaviour changes in men, particularly around sensitive topics (Robertson et al., 2008).

## CHAPTER 14

# WHAT SOME WOMEN WISH MEN KNEW

*Disclaimer: This chapter is not intended to generalise or stereotype men. It reflects the voices and lived experiences of women who have shared with me their struggles to feel heard, supported, or acknowledged in their fertility journeys. These stories deserve space – not as blame, but as insight.*

I was incredibly fortunate throughout my infertility journey. Yes, I faced loss, miscarriages, fear, and frustration. But through it all, Jordan was there – showing up, even when he didn't always have the answers. This chapter isn't just about me; it's about the importance of partners showing up in their own ways, whether it's through understanding, comfort, or sharing responsibility. This journey isn't just about reproduction; it's about making sure men are part of the conversation from the start.

Like any couple, we've had our ups and downs (definitely more ups). But what got us through wasn't perfect timing or divine luck. It was this: talking.

I never sat on my stress. I voiced it. When I felt dismissed, overwhelmed, or hurt, I said it. And Jordan did the same. Communication wasn't just about addressing the tension between us – it was about ensuring we were both present and engaged in the process of fertility, health, and emotional support. This open dialogue wasn't just about solving issues, it was about proactively protecting our relationship and our wellbeing, both of which would lay the foundation for a future with children. That communication built our connection.

And that connection? It got us through infertility.

Not just with one child, but two.

Not just with one business, but two – and now a third.

But more than anything, it gave me a partner who doesn't just support me – he lifts me.

That's the real gift our conception journey gave us – not just the children we longed for, but the *relationship* that could hold them.

And I know, painfully, that many couples don't come out the other side like we did.

I don't believe that's because they didn't love each other. I believe it's because somewhere in the heartbreak they stopped talking.

They avoided hard conversations. Or spoke at the wrong time. Or turned away instead of turning toward.

And by the time the child came (if the child came), there was so much unspoken grief and blame between them that there was nothing left to build on.

Even couples who stay together – for the kids, for appearances – often begin modelling tension. Conflict. Silence.

Kids grow up thinking this is normal. That withdrawal is love. That frustration is connection.

But we can't raise emotionally healthy kids in a house where emotional connection has gone silent.

As Cool Beans reached more people, I started hearing from others too – mostly women. Their stories were raw and familiar, filled with the grief I too had experienced, but with a crucial difference: they felt as though they had carried the burden of infertility alone. But many men also carry this burden, though in silence, while they support their partners. Without solutions or knowing how to be actively involved in improving their conception outcomes, men are largely left as bystanders. And while we may think that men need to show up more – not only physically but emotionally – maybe it's time we open conversations and undertake fertility responsibilities together. Since launching Cool Beans, I've received dozens of messages from women who feel completely lost asking how to get their partners more involved – often too scared that it will sound accusatory.

They're desperate to have conversations with their partners about fertility, hormone health, sperm, testing. But they don't know how.

Some write to ask, "How do I talk to him about this without making him feel blamed?"

Others are scared. "I want to buy him some Cool Beans, but I'm worried he'll take it the wrong way."

They've already done everything. Changed their diets. Tracked their cycles. Taken supplements. Had bloodwork. Ultrasounds. Surgeries.

And their partner still hasn't even done a sperm test. How can they convince their husband and partners to be proactive and not dismissive?

They're exhausted. Not just by the process – but by the emotional load of having to carry it *alone*.

This is where so many relationships begin to crumble. Fortunately, this isn't the case for all – but it is for far too many and until we can normalise the men's health conversation it will continue to be this way.

Because the heartbreak of infertility is one thing. But the heartbreak of going through it alone – next to someone who won't engage – is something else entirely.

Cool Beans has become more than just a product in these moments; it's become a symbol. A way for men to show up in ways they may not have known how to before. It's a gesture that says: *'I love you. I see you. I'm here with you.'* By taking this step, men are saying they're willing to be a part of the solution – whether it's fertility, emotional support, or simply showing they care.

For some couples, Cool Beans is the first time the man takes action. The first time the woman doesn't have to chase, explain, or plead. It's not invasive. It doesn't threaten ego. It doesn't require words.

It just arrives in a package.

And that's enough to change everything.

To be clear, we have an incredibly high male customer rate. Many of our customers are men who found us themselves, who wanted to be proactive, who wanted something they could do *now* – to be involved.

And that's not a contradiction. It's a reflection of diversity.

Some men are ready. Some aren't. Some relationships have open dialogue. Others don't. Some women feel empowered to speak freely. Others are carrying layers of grief, shame, or cultural silence.

And across all of it, there's one clear truth: women are often the ones pushing for change.

They are the ones researching. Initiating. Holding hope.

What women wish men knew isn't just about sperm health, it's about showing up for the full journey. It's about being fully engaged – openly and consistently. Men, take part in the emotional and physical aspects of fertility. Be proactive. Get tested. Don't wait for things to fall apart before you act. Men's fertility health is integral to this journey, and when they show up, it makes all the difference in the outcome.

It's about partnership.

About how lonely it feels when you're the only one fighting for the family.

About how painful it is to feel like you're trying to force someone to care.

About how devastating it is to go through loss and feel like you must manage your grief *and* protect his.

What women wish men knew is that their silence doesn't shield them. It hurts them. This chapter isn't about blame. It's about balance. And what it feels like when one person is carrying it all, quietly hoping the other will meet them there.

That doing nothing *is* doing something – but is that how you want to show up?

And that the simplest gestures – a test, a pair of underwear, a conversation – can be the difference between growing together or growing apart. What women wish men knew is that showing up doesn't need to be perfect, it just needs to be real. Sometimes, taking that first step in the journey – whether it's buying a pair of Cool Beans, having an open conversation, or getting tested – is the most meaningful way to show you care. It's a way to actively engage, to say *'I'm here, I'm involved, and I want to be part of this.'* Men – don't wait. Your proactive action could be the difference between a struggle and a shared success.

This chapter was the turning point for me. Not just in the mission. But in the book.

Cool Beans wasn't just about male fertility anymore.

It was about emotional load. Communication. Culture. Relationships. Healing.

It was about women.

And what they carry.

And why they shouldn't have to carry it alone.

While cultural, social, and individual contexts vary worldwide, the underlying emotional needs remain universal. Whether single, partnered, LGBTQ+, or blended, every journey deserves visibility, empathy, and genuine partnership.

## Putting it into practice

**For him** – Your support is more than just physical – it's emotional too.

- Show up emotionally, not just physically:
    - Ask your partner how she's really doing – not just during appointments, but in the quiet in-between moments. Let her see you care.
    - Being emotionally available and engaged helps her feel safe, supported, and less alone in the process.
    - Emotional availability in male partners has been linked to reduced stress and improved relationship satisfaction in couples facing infertility (Martins et al., 2014).
- Be proactive in your fertility journey:
    - Get a sperm test early. Wear garments similar to Cool Beans. Reduce daily heat exposure. Take accountability for your part of the equation.
    - Fertility is a shared journey – and sperm health contributes to nearly half of conception outcomes.
    - Male factor infertility is involved in 50% of cases, yet often goes untested or untreated (Agarwal et al., 2015).

**For her** – This journey isn't yours to carry alone – ask for the support you need and share the load.

- Share your emotional needs clearly and regularly:
    - Let your partner know what kind of support helps most – whether that's physical, verbal, or shared planning.
    - When you express your needs directly, it prevents resentment and improves connection.
    - Open communication improves couple resilience and outcomes in fertility-related stress (Pasch & Sullivan, 2017).
- Release the belief that you have to carry it all alone:
    - Ask for help. Share the load. Let your partner step up – even if it's imperfect.
    - Shared emotional labour prevents burnout and strengthens long-term relationship health.
    - Uneven distribution of emotional and logistical fertility labour is linked to psychological strain in female partners (Greil et al., 2011).

**For us** – This is a shared journey – one of both emotional and physical connection.

- Turn toward each other, not away:
    - Make space for each other's fears, grief, and dreams – without judgment or silence.
    - Emotional responsiveness is one of the strongest predictors of long-term relationship strength and post-infertility growth.
    - Couples who engage in shared meaning-making and supportive dialogue have higher relationship satisfaction and lower distress during fertility treatment (Peterson et al., 2006).
- Create rituals of connection that go beyond fertility:
    - Take walks. Share meals. Talk about something other than cycles and test results. Reconnect as people – not just as parents-in-waiting.

CoolBeans

- o These moments build intimacy and resilience, which will carry you into parenthood and beyond.
- o Maintaining non-fertility-focused intimacy helps protect against emotional burnout and preserves relationship identity (Leiblum, 2001).

## Behind the chapter: Sources

- Women undergoing infertility treatment report emotional distress levels comparable to patients with cancer or heart disease (Domar et al., 1993).
- When male partners are untested or disengaged, women experience significantly higher levels of anxiety and resentment (Greil et al., 2011).
- Couples who communicate openly about fertility challenges are more likely to maintain relationship satisfaction and successfully adapt post-treatment (Peterson et al., 2006).
- Shared participation in fertility planning improves emotional closeness and coping ability (Martins et al., 2014).
- Perceived imbalance in fertility responsibility leads to higher rates of emotional exhaustion and relational conflict (Pasch & Sullivan, 2017).

## CHAPTER 15
# WHAT MEN WISH THEY COULD SAY

I've read countless messages from men that start with some version of, *'I've never told anyone this before...'*. These aren't just messages about sperm health. They're messages about pain – physical, emotional – and the kind of pain many have carried silently. Men have been trained to mask discomfort, to dismiss emotions, and to carry burdens without question.

Sometimes it's about fertility. Sometimes it's about shame. Sometimes it's about pain – physical or emotional. Pain, they have carried for years – in silence.

And more often than not, the message comes after they've tried Cool Beans.

There's something about the act of wearing something that was designed specifically for them – not just for fashion or function, but for health, for comfort, for care – that opens a door to conversation.

They realise they've been overlooked. Not intentionally. But historically. For so long, male fertility wasn't part of the conversation – not in research, not in treatment. It wasn't until the 1980s that male factor infertility was even formally recognised. And around the same time, male fertility began its global decline.

The system isn't against men – it's just grown used to their silence. It has adapted to their absence. And so have many of them.

This is the essence of emotional vulnerability – a space that society has long closed off for men. Vulnerability isn't about weakness; it's the doorway to better health, stronger relationships, and true connection. It's about breaking cycles of silence and embracing the idea that real strength comes from being seen and understood, not from hiding.

Many of these men don't have the words. Not because they're incapable – but because no one ever handed them the language.

They were taught to endure. To provide. To tough it out. To keep it together.

So they didn't say anything when they felt pain after surgery. They didn't speak up when sex didn't feel the same. They didn't ask questions when they and their partner couldn't conceive. They just... carried it.

And when Cool Beans arrived? Suddenly, someone had thought about *them*. Not about their productivity. Not about their strength. But their softness. Their biology. Their wellbeing.

Cool Beans Underwear® became a quiet yes.

This isn't just about comfort or fertility; it's about letting men know they're worth caring for, not just for their productivity or strength but for their biological and emotional wellbeing. The act of taking care of one's health, of addressing discomfort – be it physical or emotional – is powerful in its simplicity. It's a tool for men to reconnect with their bodies, their emotions, and their partners.

Not all men are silent. Some are emotionally fluent, expressive, proactive. But too many aren't – not because they don't want to be, but because they were never given the tools. They weren't raised with the language, or the space, or the permission. And when it comes to sperm health, many men shut down completely. They fear what it might say

# What men wish they could say

about their masculinity. About their worth. They fear blame, shame, or the possibility that they are the reason things aren't working – even when their partner never once said that.

So instead of engaging, some dismiss. Some deflect. Some stay silent – not out of arrogance, but out of fear.

And when you see it for what it is – not pride, but protection – you start to understand the walls men build around their vulnerability aren't meant to keep you out. They're just all they've ever known.

I never expected that.

I knew we were building something for sperm health. For testicular function. For temperature and recovery.

But I didn't know we were building something that would let men say, *"I've never felt anything like this before – and not just physically."*

That's the power of intention.

When you design something with care, care becomes contagious.

One man wrote:

> "I honestly thought I was broken. We'd tried everything. When I saw your product, I figured it was for guys who were already further down the track. But I gave it a go. And when I put them on, I realised just how much tension I'd been carrying around for years without noticing. It felt like something shifted."

Another:

> "I'd had this dull, annoying pain for years. It never really went away – just became something I put up with. I tried a bunch of things. Physio. Acupuncture. Even surgery. But nothing really worked. A mate mentioned Cool Beans, and I figured why not. I don't know exactly why, but something about them just helped. I actually sit comfortably now. It's the first thing that's made a difference."

These aren't product reviews. These are confessions. Gratitude. Letters from men who finally feel *understood*.

And what I've learned is this: men don't need a miracle. They just need permission. To soften. To speak. To feel. To be something other than the strong one.

What do men wish they could say? I'm scared. I'm tired. I don't know what's wrong. I feel like I'm failing. I don't want to let her down. I wish someone would ask about me for once. I wish I didn't have to be strong all the time. I wish I knew how to fix this. I wish I could say it without shame. Not perfection. Not performance. Just presence.

And when men feel that invitation – without judgment or pressure – they show up. They show up beautifully.

Which brings me to Jordan.

He is many things: my partner, my co-founder, the first model for Cool Beans, the man I've raised two children with, and the person who – when I wanted to give up – reminded me why I started.

But one thing he isn't? A big talker.

Jordan doesn't do long speeches. He doesn't share his feelings in poetic paragraphs. But he feels deeply. And he shows it.

This speaks to the broader reality many men face: the quiet ways they show up when the world tells them to remain stoic. A simple act, like wearing Cool Beans, can open the door to deeper conversations, less about the product and more about the internal shifts that allow men to step into their emotional health. Men don't always need words – sometimes it's about the quiet, consistent action that sparks bigger changes.

Every late-night prototype he wore without complaint. Every time he tested a new design and gave quiet, detailed feedback. Every time he believed in this mission when it was still just an idea.

That was his way of speaking.

## What men wish they could say

He doesn't need to say much. He never has. But his actions – wearing the first samples when we were still grieving, turning up to trade shows, quality checking samples with a ruler in one hand and a toddler in the other – that's always been how Jordan shows up. Quietly. Fully.

That's what makes his support matter. Not because it's loud, but because it's constant.

> "What stands out to me in this chapter isn't just the product or the process, it's what sits underneath it all. Most men don't talk about this stuff. They've been taught to tough it out, to keep quiet, and to just get on with it. So, when something as simple as a pair of underwear gives them a reason to open up – even a little – it matters. It's not really about fabric or design; it's about telling men, maybe for the first time, that they're allowed to care about themselves, too. That it's okay to ask questions, to admit fear, to feel disappointed or hopeful. And in my case, it wasn't speeches that did it. It was small, practical steps, researching, testing, wearing the prototypes, even when I didn't know if it would help. Sometimes that's all it takes: a small, deliberate act that says, 'You matter too.' And that can open a door that men didn't know they were waiting for."
> – Jordan

And I think a lot of men feel the same way.

They're waiting for someone to see them. To say, *"You matter. Your health matters. Your voice matters."*

Cool Beans may have started with science. But it's ending with something deeper.

If you're reading this and feel like something inside you is stirring – that's the voice you've been told to ignore. Please don't. Let this be your yes. A yes to comfort. A yes to care. A yes to being seen.

This chapter is not just about what men wish they could say. It's about what they *do* say – when we finally make space for them to be heard.

And this is what the book is about: creating a space where men can speak freely. Where the silence around their health, their emotions, and their fears is finally broken. Men deserve to show up for themselves, to acknowledge their struggles, and to feel supported. Cool Beans is just a product. The real change is in the culture we create around it. A culture that allows men to be seen as they are, without judgment, without silence.

> *"When Saara made that first prototype, the one I wore every day for months – I didn't know if it would actually help. But we had nothing to lose. I didn't say much at the time, but part of me worried it wouldn't make any difference. That it'd end up meaning nothing. But after a few months, something did change. And we conceived. I still don't talk about it much, but looking back, I'm glad I wore them. I'm proud of Saara. And I'm proud that what we made helps other guys feel like they're not alone – that what they're going through is real and recognised."*
> *– Jordan*

## Putting it into practice

**For him** – Your actions speak louder than words: show up for yourself and for those you love.

- Join a men's health group or even just a BBQ where real talk is on the table:
    - Whether it's catching up with mates or joining a casual community group, surround yourself with other men who aren't afraid to talk about what's really going on.

- - Being around emotionally open men helps break the pattern of silence.
  - Peer support groups have been shown to reduce psychological distress and improve health-seeking behaviour among men (Robertson et al., 2013).
- Choose one area of discomfort and address it:
  - Whether it's testicular pain, fatigue, or mood, take one small action to improve it – book a check-up, switch your underwear, or have a conversation.
  - Health starts when we stop ignoring what's easy to tolerate.
  - Men who take early action on symptoms experience better treatment outcomes and fewer complications (Banks et al., 2014).

**For her** – Your support doesn't need to be perfect, just present and understanding.

- Ask how he's feeling – but also prepare for silence, shutdown, or resistance:
  - If he avoids the topic or shuts it down completely, don't take it personally. Try again later – with curiosity, not pressure. Suggest a podcast, hand him a pair of Cool Beans, or leave an article open. Your job isn't to force the conversation – just to keep inviting it.
  - Many men have gone their whole lives without safe permission to talk about these things – sometimes they need to see it modelled first.
  - Exposure to indirect, low-pressure prompts can help emotionally avoidant men engage over time (Seidler et al., 2016).
- Recognise and affirm the quiet efforts:
  - If he starts showing up in small ways – wearing Cool Beans, reading an article, making a change – let him know you see it.
  - These acknowledgements build trust and momentum.

- Positive reinforcement is one of the strongest predictors of sustained behavioural change in couples (Heyman, 2001).

**For us** – Strengthen your bond by facing challenges together.

- Create micro-moments of connection that aren't about performance:
  - Sit together. Eat together. Check in. No agenda. No tasks. Just presence.
  - It's in these quiet moments that emotional intimacy grows.
  - Everyday connection rituals increase couple resilience during stressful life events (Gottman & Silver, 1999).
- Challenge outdated ideas of masculinity – together:
  - Talk about what strength actually looks like in your home. Let boys and men be tender, uncertain, or tired – and know that it's safe.
  - Culture shifts when couples model a new way of being.
  - Redefining masculine norms around emotional expression leads to better mental health outcomes for men and stronger family dynamics (Seidler et al., 2016).

## Behind the chapter: Sources

- Men are significantly less likely to seek help for health concerns, often delaying treatment until symptoms are severe (Addis & Mahalik, 2003).
- Male infertility is involved in up to 50% of conception issues but remains under-discussed and under-tested (Agarwal et al., 2015).
- Cultural pressure to 'man up' leads to emotional suppression, poor mental health, and weakened relationship communication (Mahalik et al., 2003).

- Small behavioural shifts, such as community connection or emotional reinforcement, dramatically improve male engagement in health (Robertson et al., 2013).
- Couples who co-create emotionally open environments model healthier behaviours for their children and experience stronger relational satisfaction (Gottman & Silver, 1999).

## THIS SIDE OF THE STORY
## – TURNING SHAME INTO POWER

Reading these stories from men – raw, anonymous, unexpected – it hits you just how much silence is sitting beneath the surface. Not just around fertility, but around pain. Discomfort. Emotions. Shame. Things so many men have been taught to ignore, deny, or bury.

That silence has a cost. And I felt it as I read through survey responses, feedback, emails and DMs. You can hear it between the lines. The quiet weight of things unsaid.

But what struck me most wasn't just the pain – it was how willing these men were to share when finally given the chance. When someone asked. When someone cared. That's when I realised: breaking this taboo doesn't just change the present. It reshapes the future. The way we talk. The way we connect. The way we raise our sons.

If we can help men start naming what they feel, what they carry, what they've normalised for far too long – we give them the tools to pass on something different. We give the next generation a new blueprint. They don't have to inherit the silence. They don't have to harden just to survive. They can grow up knowing that true strength includes vulnerability. That masculinity isn't about closing off, it's about showing up and embracing the fullness of who they are, without shame.

They don't have to inherit the silence. They don't have to harden just to survive. They can grow up knowing that real strength includes softness. That masculinity isn't about closing off – it's about showing up.

And it starts with us. With you. With me. With all of us learning how to sit with our own discomfort long enough to let someone else feel safe in theirs.

That's what these stories gave me. Not just perspective. But purpose. We aren't just healing men. We're shaping fathers. And through them, shaping a new world, one where men can thrive emotionally, physically, and relationally.

This shift requires all of us. Men and women, partners and allies, individuals and communities. It's time to break old silences, confront shame with understanding, and rewrite the narrative together, because when we heal men, we heal families and future generations.

**CoolBeans**

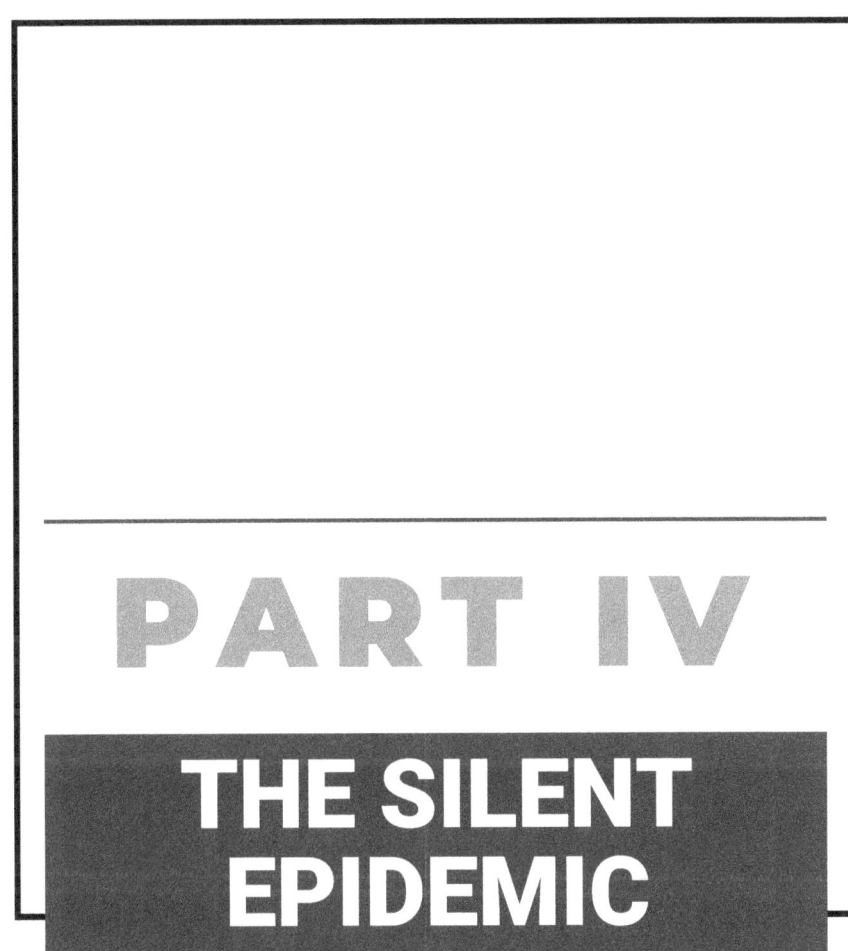

# PART IV
# THE SILENT EPIDEMIC

**CoolBeans**

## CHAPTER 16
# THE COST OF VISION

If you've made it this far, thank you. Not just for reading, but for braving the discomfort alongside me, navigating hard truths, complicated science, and layers of grief we seldom speak aloud. This next part isn't merely about biology. It's about breaking silences. It's about reclaiming identity. It's about confronting systems that were never built to carry the invisible burdens of men's pain.

Cool Beans was never just underwear. It was always about something bigger. A movement. A reckoning. A response to the silence that so many men carry – and the women who carry it beside them.

Let me be blunt: bringing a first-of-its-kind medical device to life without external investment nearly broke us. There was no runway. No safety net. We made it work, but not without cost.

Jordan has had to take quiet cash advances on his pay, those insidious quick fixes that creep up on you, slowly eroding your credit rating without you noticing. We didn't fully grasp the impact until reality knocked on our door, demanding a personal loan to place our first batch of manufacturing, and leaving us stalled for three more anxious months, waiting, worrying, hoping.

Eventually, we secured a loan to cover manufacturing costs that allowed us to finally launch and enter the market. That's the thing with product-based businesses: the requirement to fund everything before ever making a dollar. Materials, design, production, packaging, shipping. All of it upfront. At this stage, despite the external validation and feedback from consumers and clinicians, we still felt like we were going in with blind faith.

I remember standing over my jewellery box one night – a small collection of necklaces, bracelets, heirlooms. I picked up my engagement ring and weighed its worth against the next import duty invoice. Jordan noticed. His gaze met mine, quiet understanding replacing words. He reached over, gently closed my hand around the ring, and whispered, "Not this one. Nothing sentimental." It was never about money; it was about the heartbeats, memories, and promises woven into precious metals and small stones.

Still, I combed through the rest of it – some of it more sentimental than others. I found a gold buyer on the north side of Brisbane. Heidi inherited the playful costume jewellery of no value. I took in a bundle of pieces, including some beautiful rings I assumed would be worth more – but tiny diamonds, even many of them, don't add up to much. They value it for parts – the weight of gold, the number and clarity of stones. I ended up selling a few that weren't too meaningful and got just enough to cover the import tax on our commercial order.

Cool Beans is now proudly manufactured in Vietnam – after a disastrous experience trying to be Australian made. We pre-launched with Australian-made stock for validation and feedback, but it didn't compare. I tried so hard with our Aussie manufacturer. I wanted to believe in him. I justified the delays, the excuses, the mistakes. I believed he was trying.

But business has a way of forcing you to see people for who they really are. And sometimes, they will use you. Fool you. Take your money and run. As it turned out, he subcontracted our production to a factory we never approved – or ever knew about – one that hadn't gone through sampling. Over 300 units came back unwearable. Worse, I'd already paid him for fabric and waistband stock to prep for our next run. That money? Gone. Used to pay off his own debts. Manufacturing wasn't just a challenge – it was a hard lesson in trust.

When we officially launched in early 2024, we had zero capital. Not to keep the business running, and not to pay our kids' school tuition. To stay afloat, I took on a full-time contract with CSIRO. Program Manager in Biosecurity Innovation. Twelve months of 100+ hour weeks. I barely saw my kids. I was already working before sunrise. Working late into the evening and often into the early morning. I remember one night crawling into bed fully clothed, too exhausted to shower, too sick to stay upright. Jordan had moved to the couch – I had a cold and was snoring too loud to sleep beside.

We made the strategic choice not to raise capital pre-launch. We knew that if we did, we'd have to give away a large chunk of our business – a business we had spent years building – for very little in return. So, I went back to corporate life to fund the gap. We are still yet to raise – we're starting to put plans into place for a future raise.

There were nights I lay awake wondering what the hell we were doing. My parents supported us by helping us with our bank loan for Cool Beans. But since then both sets of parents, mine and Jordan's, have supported us in numerous ways to aid us in our mission. Every type of support, no matter how big or little, whether it was financial or looking after the kids, came as life-changing support that was enough to keep the wheels turning. Enough to say: 'We believe in you.'

And honestly, sometimes that belief was the only thing that kept us going. When the numbers didn't add up and the doubt crept in, their quiet confidence became our cushion.

Building a business from scratch isn't just lonely, it's misunderstood. Especially by those who've never had to risk everything. What you sacrifice isn't just time or sleep, it's certainty. It's school tuition, loan repayments, and making sure you can still put food on the table. Not having the reliability of a constant salary or even regular sales in the early days and having chosen not to bring on investment too early on – we were sacrificing everything.

Cool Beans wasn't a side hustle. It began as our answer to infertility, to years of medical gaslighting and missing science. It was the hope that no other couple would have to go through what we did without a tool that could've changed the outcome. That kind of mission isn't small or finite – and so it's grown beyond underwear into a broader mission for men's health, a tool for protecting fertility, supporting hormone balance, and improving wellbeing at every stage of life.

And when you're in the middle of that pressure, when the balance sheet is inches from collapse, stepping away, even for a weekend, isn't a break. It's a gamble.

Yet unless someone's lived it – either the business or the infertility – they won't see that. They'll assume indifference, or worse, laziness. They won't call to ask. They won't question their assumptions. They'll decide you're absent by choice, not survival. That hurts. Because you'd give anything to show up. But right now, showing up here, holding this thing together by the seams, is the only way to protect the future you're working toward – whether that's for your children, the family you hope to have, or the people who depend on you and honour the journey that brought you to this point.

Those with financial security can step away without risking collapse. Not everyone can. And it's not about work ethic, it's about consequences. Some of us don't have the luxury of pausing. We keep working because if we don't, everything we've built, from healing to hope to purpose, will disappear.

My family has always joked about something called the 'Jelekainen Luck', a curious cocktail of near-misses, miraculous saves, and inexplicable fortunes. My brother Ari attracted free upgrades and last-second escapes. My mum survived adventures and misadventures

## The cost of vision

enough for several lifetimes. I used to believe it had skipped me entirely, until I realised my version wasn't flashy miracles, it was quiet reprieves. Shipment clearances that saved our bank account, pre-orders appearing precisely when fees came due, delayed invoices that arrived exactly when our funds hit zero. It wasn't spectacular, but it was just enough, and sometimes, just enough is everything.

When I look back on those years, I don't just see hustle. I see survival. I see what it took to hold a vision that nobody else could see yet. I see the cost of being early – too early – in a world not built for female founders talking about male anatomy.

This chapter isn't just about what we built. It's about what we were up against.

That night on the kitchen floor, sobbing at 2 am, cracked something wide open, not just within me, but between us. The walls we'd silently built to protect each other crumbled in that shared embrace. My vulnerability wasn't weakness; it was honesty. And in that honesty, Jordan found permission to lay down his silence too. Our breakdown became our breakthrough.

For too long, masculinity has been tied to silence. To pushing through. To burying pain instead of speaking it. Jordan lived this. So did our dads. So do most men we know. But what if that quiet endurance isn't strength? What if it's self-sabotage?

We're not just fighting biology. We're fighting culture. And every time we challenge these norms, we're also teaching the next generation – our sons, our daughters, our nieces and nephews – that health and emotional honesty are strengths worth protecting. A culture that mocks vulnerability. That laughs at self-care. That defaults to 'her problem' when a couple struggles to conceive.

I know because I lived every exhausting test, invasive drug, and misplaced blame. But now I see clearly that Jordan lived it too, invisibly, silently bearing the burden of helplessness beside me. Society's easy dismissal of male struggles forced him into quiet resilience. I remember a particular night coming home wrecked from work, finding him alone folding towels, jaw tense and eyes averted. "I don't want to be the reason you break," he'd whispered, quiet desperation etched in his voice. Those words, heavy with unseen pain, haunt me still.

We need a new story. One that reclaims health as strength. One that empowers men to act before they hit rock bottom. One that recognises sperm health not just as a fertility marker but as a sign of overall wellbeing.

This is for every man who's been told to harden up. For every woman who's carried the weight alone. For every couple who's been told to 'just relax' or 'just do IVF'.

We can do better. We must. Because rewriting the male narrative isn't just about men.

It's about all of us and about the children who will grow up in a world shaped by the choices we make today. We can either pass down silence and stigma or show them what it looks like to speak up, care for our health, and support others in doing the same. About breaking the silence not just for our partners, but for our sons, our daughters, and everyone who has ever sat in a waiting room alone and blamed themselves.

If we genuinely wish to rewrite our future, to free our sons and daughters from these invisible burdens and inherited silences, we must start rewriting our stories today. It begins in our homes, our conversations, and our courage. Let's choose vulnerability over silence, honesty over shame, and mutual strength over solitary suffering. Because changing the narrative isn't merely a choice, it's our responsibility. Every conversation we start, every healthy habit we model, becomes part of the foundation our children and the children around us build on as they grow into adulthood.

## Putting it into practice

**For him** – Your health is your legacy.

- Check your waistline, not just your weight:
    - Measure your waist circumference and aim to keep it under 94 cm.
    - Abdominal fat gain is linked to hormonal disruption, insulin resistance, and reduced sperm quality.
    - Men with waist circumferences over 94 cm have a higher risk of low testosterone and impaired fertility (Jensen et al., 2004).
- Protect your sleep as seriously as your training:
    - Set a consistent bedtime, reduce late-night screen time, and aim for 7–8 hours of quality sleep.
    - Poor sleep disrupts testosterone production and impairs sperm count and motility.
    - Sleeping fewer than 6 hours per night is linked to a 31% lower sperm count and poorer motility (Chen et al., 2016).
- Cool down after high-heat exposure:
    - After saunas, hot baths, or long cycling sessions, use targeted cooling (like a cold shower or cooling device) to help sperm recovery.
    - Excessive heat can impair sperm quality for weeks, but prompt cooling supports recovery.
    - Hot water immersion or prolonged scrotal heat reduces sperm motility, with recovery taking up to 3 months (Jung et al., 2001).
- Get your vitamin K2 levels checked:
    - Request a blood test for vitamin K2 and supplement if deficient under medical guidance.
    - Vitamin K2 supports healthy testosterone production and sperm motility.
    - Deficiency is linked to impaired testosterone synthesis and reduced sperm motility in men (Ito et al., 2011).

**For her** – Fertility is a full-body indicator.

- Check your iron stores before trying to conceive:
    - Ask your doctor for a ferritin test and address low levels before pregnancy.
    - Iron deficiency can delay ovulation and reduce implantation rates.
    - Women with low ferritin, even without anaemia, may experience reduced fertility (Acharya et al., 2018).
- Optimise thyroid health early:
    - Request a full thyroid panel (TSH, T3, T4, and thyroid antibodies) before conception.
    - Even mild hypothyroidism can impair fertility and increase miscarriage risk.
    - Treating borderline hypothyroidism improves conception and pregnancy outcomes (Poppe et al., 2002).
- Include resistance training:
    - Incorporate strength training into your weekly routine, aiming for 2–3 sessions.
    - Improves insulin sensitivity, hormone balance, and egg quality.
    - Resistance training is linked to improved ovulation and reproductive outcomes in women (De Souza et al., 2003).

**For us** – Shared action is stronger action.

- Have a heat-neutral home:
    - Keep laptops off laps, avoid heated blankets, and choose breathable bedding.
    - Everyday environmental heat can impair sperm quality and sleep quality for both partners.
    - Continuous low-level heat exposure can disrupt sperm production and hormone regulation (Mieusset & Bujan, 1995).

- Share stress-reduction rituals:
  - Schedule regular activities like walking, stretching, or mindfulness that you do together.
  - Shared relaxation builds emotional resilience and improves relationship satisfaction.
  - Couples who relax together report higher conception rates and stronger relationship bonds (Li et al., 2016).
- Do a joint medication and supplement audit:
  - Review all prescription, over-the-counter, and herbal products with a healthcare professional.
  - Some medications and supplements can support one partner while harming the other's fertility.
  - Certain common medications, such as NSAIDs, can impair ovulation or sperm quality (Crawford et al., 2015).

**For our children** – Building future-ready health habits.

- Teach them the value of outdoor movement:
  - Replace one hour of screen time per week with an active, outdoor family activity.
  - Builds physical resilience, supports healthy hormone regulation, and strengthens family bonds.
  - Outdoor play is linked to better cardiovascular health, lower obesity risk, and improved mood in children (Gray et al., 2015).
- Normalise conversations about body health:
  - Use everyday moments to talk about sleep, food, and activity in positive, non-judgemental ways.
  - Encourages self-awareness and lays the foundation for lifelong health habits.
  - Children who receive open health education from parents are more likely to adopt healthy behaviours into adulthood (Sonneville et al., 2012).

- Model device boundaries:
  - Have a set 'tech-free' meal or evening each week where the whole family disconnects.
  - Reduces passive screen time, improves communication skills, and supports mental wellbeing.
  - Families who eat together without devices report higher emotional connection and healthier eating habits (Fiese et al., 2012).

## Behind the Chapter: Sources

- Male factors contribute to up to 50% of infertility cases, yet most treatment still begins with the woman, delaying correct diagnosis and wasting time, money, and emotional energy (Agarwal et al., 2015).

- Declining sperm quality is linked with increased chronic disease risk, metabolic dysfunction, and shorter lifespan – making sperm health a key biomarker for long-term health, not just fertility (Eisenberg et al., 2014).

- Low testosterone is associated with fatigue, depression, reduced libido, impaired sperm production, and poorer metabolic function (Basaria, 2014).

- Chronic stress suppresses the hypothalamic-pituitary-gonadal axis, disrupting hormone signalling, reducing sperm production in men, and impairing ovulation in women (Li et al., 2011).

- Mitochondrial function directly impacts egg quality, embryo development, and implantation success – nutrients such as CoQ10 can help improve oocyte mitochondrial health (Bentov et al., 2014).

- Micronutrient deficiencies, particularly folate, B12, and vitamin D, can impair hormone balance and conception outcomes in women (Gaskins et al., 2014).

- Couples who approach fertility as a shared responsibility report lower stress, greater emotional resilience, and better decision-making during treatment (Peterson et al., 2006).
- Cultural norms that frame masculinity as emotional suppression lead to delayed medical care and poorer health outcomes for men (Courtenay, 2000).

# CoolBeans

# CHAPTER 17
# RAISING STRONGER SONS

My life changed on 21 June 2017 – the evening before I was induced. My due date was still another few weeks off, but my baby was measuring abnormally large. I had dreamed of a natural birth. I wanted to experience the full magic of life emerging from me. So, in I went to the hospital – the evening before – for the gel, the check-ins, the waiting.

I wouldn't say that an induction is without discomfort. I couldn't sleep, too wired by the anticipation of meeting our child. The following day, my vulva was on fire – swollen, throbbing, tender. They say the best way to support an induction is to walk. So, I walked and walked. Around the hospital. Through quiet corridors and back stairwells I'd never noticed before. Through the gardens until my scheduled appointment with my OBGYN at noon. I just had to make it that far.

After assessing me, they decided it was time to break my waters – my cervix had begun to dilate and was 1.5 cm. For those unfamiliar, inductions begin with prostaglandin gel; it's applied high into the vaginal canal to soften the cervix. Then, if labour doesn't start naturally, your doctor will manually rupture the membranes with an amnihook – a small tool designed to simulate the natural water breaking. The pressure. The pain. The release. I clutched the nurse's hand as she whispered, "It's almost over, just hold on a little longer."

My body responded – contractions started and built with intensity over the coming hours. They were strong. Powerful. But my cervix refused to open. After hours of effort, we made the call. Emergency C-section.

Here's the thing about me – people who know me would say I'm pretty cool, calm and collected in most scenarios. But I suppose many women wouldn't be, when they're being prepped for surgery. That day, the ward had an unprecedented number of caesareans. I was the sixth. As I was wheeled into theatre, a woman – I still don't know if she was a nurse or support staff – placed her hands on my shoulders, pressed her forehead gently to mine and whispered, "It's okay. Just breathe. They're preparing the spinal tap."

I didn't need reassurance. I wasn't panicked. But apparently, my stillness read as fear. I tried to explain I was fine, but then my OBGYN walked in – someone I'd been seeing for over two years throughout my conception journey. He glanced at me, smiled, and turned to the nurse. "She's okay. She'll be the easiest patient we have today." And just like that, the tension lifted.

I trusted him. I trusted Jordan, who was beside me the whole time. I was ready.

What I wasn't ready for was the rule that you can't watch your own surgery unless you've filed prior paperwork and signed special waivers. I'd wanted to witness every moment. But rules were rules. The curtain stayed up. I was informed that this was quite an unusual request – to want to watch your own surgery. Jordan agreed.

And then, after what felt like only a couple of minutes – the tugging, the pressure, the wait – there it was. A cry. My baby's cry.

The paediatrician held him up. A boy. A boy who promptly peed all over him. Jordan stood, eyes wide, and cut the cord. He was weighed, checked, assessed. They brought him to me and placed him on my chest while they stitched me up and the nurse asked, "Do you have a name yet?"

"Van McLeod Jamieson," I replied as tears fell down my cheeks.

He was long – 52 cm from head to toe. The original concern had been his size – projected at over 4 kg, had we waited until full term. But because we delivered early, he hadn't had time to bulk up. Van ended up only weighing 3.425 kg.

He was perfect – a little cone-headed from pushing against an unopened cervix, but that would settle over the next coming days.

Van had a touch of jaundice when he was first born, so the paediatric team moved him to the NICU, thankfully for only a few hours, for monitoring under phototherapy lights. I only had a few minutes with him before they whisked him away. Jordan went with him, and when I was finally stitched up, I met up with Jordan in the hallway. The nurse gave me a photo and said that they'd bring Van to our room shortly.

That night, I was beyond exhausted. I hadn't slept the night before, and yet I couldn't sleep until I had Van again in my arms. I placed Van onto my breast, the skin-to-skin contact calming us both, and I drifted into an exhausted sleep while Jordan watched over us and kept one eye on State of Origin Game 3.

For those not from Australia, State of Origin is one of the country's most fiercely contested rugby league competitions – a best-of-three showdown between Queensland and New South Wales that stirs deep tribal loyalty. It's intense. Tribal. Generational. And that night, in the dim glow of hospital lights, The Maroons (QLD) claimed victory.

I felt an overwhelming peace, as if something deep inside me had finally been restored after years of longing. For years, we had longed for this child. And now, here he was – breathing, warm, real.

We named him Van, after Van Morrison. It was the name I'd always known I would use. Our first wedding dance had been to *Into the Mystic*. Now, here we were again, Van Morrison playing softly in the background, Van nestled against my chest. It felt full circle.

But the world we were welcoming him into hadn't changed – yet.

As I held Van, I realised I wasn't just raising a child. I was raising a future man. A man who would inherit the choices we make today, about health, about hormones, about what masculinity even means.

He deserved a narrative better than stoicism. He deserved tools I never had access to: the science, the language, the permission to be whole.

And that was when a new thought quietly settled in.

How do I raise this boy?

Not just how do I keep him alive. But how do I raise him to thrive in a world that is so often unkind to men's health, to their emotions, to their bodies? How do I raise a strong, capable, independent boy who is also kind, body-aware, and emotionally literate?

Because here's the truth: we're failing boys. We don't prepare them for puberty like we do girls. We don't talk to them about fertility, or mental health, or the signals their body sends when something's wrong. We tell them to toughen up. Harden up. To push through. But the weight of silence is crushing them. And that silence? It gets inherited.

We don't just raise boys in our homes. We raise them in our schools, our clinics, our jokes. We raise them every time we roll our eyes when they cry or say *man up* when they're in pain.

If we don't challenge this story, they grow into men who are praised for endurance but punished for expression. Men who show up to fertility clinics twenty years too late, confused and ashamed.

Rewriting that story starts here: not in crisis, but in childhood.

If we don't speak up now, our sons will grow up thinking that pain is weakness, that crying is shameful, and that asking for help means you've failed.

Van will grow up knowing what sperm is – he already does. What testosterone does. How sleep, stress, movement, and even underwear, can affect his body. He'll know that his emotions aren't liabilities – they're data. He'll know that rest is strength. That resilience isn't about holding it in – it's about knowing when to let it out.

Raising stronger sons means more than protecting their physical health. It's teaching them the language of their body and giving them permission to use it. It means teaching them that masculinity is not one thing. It's many things – and it evolves. It's strength and softness. Courage and care. Curiosity and calm. It's also messy and imperfect. That's the beauty of it.

I want Van to grow up knowing that his body isn't something to ignore, override, or be ashamed of. It's something to respect. To listen to. I want him to understand how hormones affect his mood, how food and sleep affect his focus, and how rest and recovery make him stronger. I want him to know that his future fertility matters too – not just for making babies, but for his entire system.

I want him to know that being a man doesn't mean suffering in silence. It means standing up for yourself. And it means standing up for others.

This chapter isn't just about Van.

It's about all our sons. About the thousands of boys being born into a world of declining health and outdated expectations. It's about what we owe them.

Not perfection. But preparation.

And you don't need a perfect plan to start. You just need to decide that silence ends with you. That one conversation, one question, one moment of honesty matters. That's how we rewrite the story – one boy, one day, one choice at a time.

Because even if you're not raising a son, you're influencing one. They're watching how we speak, how we show up, how we rest, how we lead. Let's show them what strong really means.

Let's raise boys who know better, so they grow into men who feel stronger – in their health, in their hearts, and in their relationships.

Because this isn't just about our sons. It's about what happens when we listen to our daughters, our partners, and our own bodies – and choose to do better.

## Putting it into practice

**For him** – Speak up and know your body.

- Learn your own health signals:
    - Use a simple health journal or app (e.g., Daylio, Apple Health) to track weekly changes in sleep, mood, weight, libido, and energy for at least three months.
    - Early signs of stress, hormone imbalance, or illness are often subtle; catching them early makes treatment easier.
    - Men who monitor their health and act quickly have better long-term outcomes (WHO, 2022).
- Normalise emotional honesty:
    - Schedule a monthly check-in with a trusted mate, partner, or counsellor – use prompts like 'One thing I'm struggling with' to start the conversation.
    - Emotional bottling increases stress and can lead to depression, anger, and relationship breakdowns.
    - Men who talk openly about feelings have lower rates of depression and anxiety (Chaplin & Aldao, 2013).

- Challenge outdated stereotypes:
  - When someone says 'man up' or 'boys don't cry', respond with a calm counter like 'Strong men share' or 'It's healthy to feel'.
  - Breaking toxic masculinity norms supports healthier behaviour and better mental health.
  - Rigid gender norms are linked to higher suicide risk and poorer relationship outcomes (WHO, 2022).

**For her** – Champion male health and openness.

- Talk about men's health as openly as women's health:
  - Once a month, ask your partner how they're feeling physically and emotionally, and listen without judgement.
  - Openness builds trust and removes stigma for your partner or male relatives.
  - Women who engage in male health discussions help men take preventive action earlier (Pluhar & Kuriloff, 2004).
- Support emotional safety:
  - When your partner shares something, repeat back what you heard – 'It sounds like you're feeling...' – before offering advice.
  - Feeling heard without judgment increases confidence and reduces stress hormones.
  - Emotional validation is linked to better coping and relationship satisfaction (Gottman et al., 1997).
- Challenge harmful cultural norms:
  - When you see unrealistic male portrayals in the media, discuss them with your partner or children and highlight healthy alternatives.
  - Awareness helps dismantle unrealistic expectations for boys and men.
  - Exposure to diverse and healthy male role models improves self-esteem and behaviour (Mahalik et al., 2003).

**For our sons** – Raise health-aware, emotionally strong boys.

Let's teach boys that knowing their bodies, owning their emotions, and asking for help is not just okay -– it's heroic.

- Teach emotional vocabulary early:
    - Play 'feelings charades' or use a feelings chart weekly to practise naming emotions.
    - Kids who can label emotions are better at self-control and decision-making.
    - Emotional literacy improves mental health and social success into adulthood (Schonert-Reichl et al., 2015).
- Explain how the male body works:
    - Use age-appropriate books or short videos to teach boys about puberty, hormones, sleep, and fertility from age 9–10.
    - This knowledge empowers boys to care for themselves before problems arise.
    - Health education in adolescence is linked to lifelong positive habits (UNESCO, 2018).
- Normalise help-seeking:
    - Share a personal story about a time you asked for help and encourage them to do the same when needed.
    - Boys who see help-seeking as strength avoid silent suffering.
    - Early help-seeking reduces the severity of mental health and physical problems (Rickwood et al., 2005).

**For us** – Create communities that support healthy boys and men.

- Create safe spaces for men and boys to talk:
    - Support or start a monthly men's group at a school, sports club, or workplace where conversations are kept confidential.
    - Safe spaces foster trust, confidence, and emotional resilience.
    - Psychological safety improves communication and problem-solving (Edmondson, 1999).

- Celebrate diverse masculinity:
  - Share stories in your family or community that celebrate empathy, creativity, and care, not just strength and competition.
  - Expanding what it means to 'be a man' protects against shame and low self-worth.
  - Acceptance of diverse traits is linked to higher wellbeing in boys and men (Mahalik et al., 2003).
- Be role models together:
  - Coordinate with other adults in a child's life (teachers, coaches, uncles) to reinforce the same healthy habits and messages.
  - Consistency across different role models reinforces values and behaviours.
  - Boys with multiple positive male role models show higher resilience and achievement (Werner & Smith, 2001).

## Behind the chapter: Sources

- 1 in 5 boys will experience a mental health disorder before the age of 18, yet early intervention and emotional openness can significantly reduce long-term risk (AIHW, 2022).
- Boys are less likely than girls to seek help for emotional issues and are often misdiagnosed due to differences in how distress presents, such as increased irritability rather than sadness (Zachrisson et al., 2006).
- Testosterone production during puberty influences not just sexual development, but also sleep patterns, emotional regulation, and brain maturation – meaning hormonal health during adolescence can have lifelong mental health implications (Sisk & Zehr, 2005).
- Health education that includes male reproductive function improves health outcomes and reduces stigma, especially when delivered early and consistently (UNESCO, 2018).

- Male suicide rates remain significantly higher than female rates in nearly all countries, with men accounting for approximately 75% of suicide deaths globally (WHO, 2021).
- Societal expectations around masculinity can lead to 'normative male alexithymia' – difficulty identifying and expressing emotions – which increases risk for depression, substance abuse, and relationship breakdowns (Levant et al., 2009).
- Men are less likely than women to seek help for mental health concerns, often delaying until symptoms become severe. Early intervention improves outcomes, yet only about 30% of men experiencing mental health problems access professional help (Mahalik et al., 2003; Addis & Mahalik, 2003).
- Adolescent boys who are taught emotional regulation skills are more likely to demonstrate resilience and reduced aggressive behaviours in adulthood (Schonert-Reichl et al., 2015).
- Positive role modelling during adolescence – especially from fathers, uncles, coaches, and teachers – significantly predicts improved mental wellbeing, reduced delinquency, and healthier adult relationships (Werner & Smith, 2001).
- Community-based male support programs, including structured peer groups, have been shown to reduce depressive symptoms and improve social connection among men of all ages (Seidler et al., 2021).

## THIS SIDE OF THE STORY
### – LETTER TO MY SON:
### WHAT STRENGTH REALLY MEANS

Today, as I wrote the last chapter, the house was full of school holiday noise, the kind that drifts in between keystrokes and makes you pause mid-thought. The kids are home. Between edits, we baked banana muffins. I stepped away to let Van take the lead with his sister, starting with cleaning the kitchen, measuring flour, and pouring batter. By the end, they'd done almost everything themselves. I couldn't believe it.

Over the weekend, Van turned eight. Still the tall kid with the cheeky grin – born at the tail-end of June, the youngest in his grade, yet somehow towering over most of his classmates. Lately, I've noticed a shift – he's not just playing anymore, he's watching. Listening. Absorbing.

He's seen what it's taken to build Cool Beans. The late nights. The tears. The way it's impacted not just me, but our family. But I think – slowly – he's beginning to understand that anything meaningful requires sacrifice. That nothing worth having comes easy. That hard work can shape something powerful.

Today, out of all days, he told me he wanted to start a business. He's mentioned it before. But today felt different. There was a look of determination in his eyes I hadn't seen before. We spent hours brainstorming – talking about impact, time, cost, meaning. We found a mission. A name. Even played around with logo ideas. It was exciting. Not because it's polished or perfect, but because of what it represents.

Because what it represents is bigger than products or logos, it's a boy learning that ideas have value. That dreams come with trade-offs. That strength can be quiet persistence, showing up again and again, even when no one else can see what you're building yet.

In a way, it's the same quiet conviction I carried when Cool Beans was just an idea, scribbled in notebooks and lived in long nights. He doesn't know it yet, but he's already walking a version of that same path. The difference is: he'll have the tools. The awareness. The language.

And maybe, one day, the world will meet a young man who never had to unlearn hiding his emotions, or learn what it means to feel.

He's learning what independence looks like. What it means to build something from nothing. What it means to chase an idea because it matters to you.

Even when he was small, he was like this. Kind. Thoughtful. Empathetic. He'd try to settle his sister when she cried. Offer cuddles when I was stressed. Use his humour or his hugs to brighten the mood of a whole room. He's always had this instinct to care, to put others first.

And now, watching that kindness evolve into purpose – I see the beginning of the man he'll one day become.

This is my side of the story – one you may not recall, but I hope you'll always feel in the man you become.

> My dearest Van,
>
> There's a lot I want to teach you in this life. But more than anything, I want you to know this:
>
> You don't have to be anyone but yourself.
>
> You don't have to carry silence as if it's strength. You don't have to pretend you're fine when you're not. You don't have to live by someone else's idea of what it means to be a man.

The world will try to tell you otherwise. It'll tell you to harden up. Push through. Stay quiet. But I want you to push back. Ask questions. Speak out. Feel everything.

Because –that is strength.

You were born from persistence. From love. From years of waiting and wondering if you'd ever arrive. And when you did, you filled a space in our hearts we didn't even know was still empty.

I didn't just create Cool Beans for our past. I created it for your future. For you to grow up in a world where men understand their bodies. Where health isn't taboo. Where rest, emotion, and vulnerability are part of the conversation.

Your body is yours to understand. Your emotions are not flaws – they're your compass. And your strength? It will never be about silence. It will be in your kindness. In your leadership. In how you stand up for others. And for yourself.

You already do that now.

I am so proud of the boy you are. But even more, I'm proud of the man you're becoming.

And I can't wait to walk beside you as you become him.

Love always,
your Mum xxxx

**CoolBeans**

## CHAPTER 18

# AND THEN CAME HEIDI

They say no two births are ever the same. If Van's arrival was marked by quiet awe and soft music, Heidi's was chaos, grit, and fire.

It began on 4 April 2019. I wasn't due until 5 May, but Heidi had other plans; or rather, my body did.

In the days leading up to her birth, life was... a lot. Van was 20 months old and keeping me on my toes. I was drowning in legal paperwork – untangling a mess left by my original IP lawyer who had missed critical deadlines and failed to meet their obligations. I was knee-deep in emails and documentation, working with a new firm to salvage our patent applications. Throughout what was to come I would need to finish off the patent applications while in hospital. I was heavily pregnant and highly stressed. And on top of it all, I had developed high blood pressure early in the pregnancy. I'd had it with Van too, but this time, I needed medication just to keep it in check.

That afternoon, I walked down to the yard where Mum was playing with Van. He ran over to me, and I picked him up – and that's when I felt something sharp pull in my side. I thought I'd strained a muscle. We went inside to rest and watch TV. But the pain didn't settle. It continued to escalate as the afternoon wore on.

I made dinner and tried to push through, but I eventually excused myself and jumped in the shower to see if the warmth might ease the pain. That's when every muscle across my lower abdomen and pelvis seized, tight as a drum. Something wasn't right.

I rang my sister-in-law, who was a midwife. She advised calling the maternity ward – and as she predicted, they told me to come in for a check-up. I was 34 weeks and five days pregnant. I was certain I'd be home in a few hours, so I didn't pack a bag – just grabbed my phone, wallet and keys.

After about an hour of monitoring, I began having early contractions. I was going into preterm labour. They gave me an injection to slow things down and told me I'd need to stay overnight for observation.

The next morning, my OBGYN walked in with a smile. "What are you doing in here?" he asked, grinning. "Causing mischief, I hear."

We laughed. Baby looked good. I looked fine too. I was due to go home that afternoon.

That was until I felt a strange sensation in my chest.

By then, my OBGYN had left for the weekend, so I was handed over to the on-call obstetrician. He didn't know me. Didn't know how I operated. I tried to explain something didn't feel right, but he waved it off.

"It must have been very scary to go into early labour," he said kindly, but very matter-of-fact as well.

"No, I don't think so," I replied. "I think something else might be going on."

He prescribed Valium and kept me overnight. But by that evening, my chest pain had intensified, and he was called back, along with the emergency team. Soon I had eight doctors crowded into my tiny hospital room, running tests, trying to work out what was happening. I had an ECG. It came back normal. I was given more Valium and Panadol – neither touched the pain.

The next morning, I was sent for a CT scan with contrast dye. I had to lie flat for the scan – something I hadn't realised would be so excruciating. It felt like someone was stabbing me in the chest. I had silent tears streaming down my face as I forced myself to stay still for the imaging.

As soon as I sat up, the pain eased slightly. But I was left shaken. What was happening to me?

Later that day, I had an echocardiogram – again, no obvious signs of heart damage. I was placed on oxygen. The Valium no longer helped. My sister-in-law came to sit with me. She stayed for hours. I could barely speak from the pain.

Finally, at 11pm, the on-call cardiologist walked in on his way home. He was seasoned and experienced – and it showed. He listened to my heart, then nodded knowingly.

"You have pericarditis," he said. "I can hear the rub."

(Pericarditis is inflammation of the membrane surrounding the heart. The 'rub' is a sound doctors can hear through a stethoscope when the inflamed layers scrape against each other with each heartbeat.) He started treatment immediately.

They gave me the highest dose of prednisone steroids they could safely administer. Within a few hours, the pain began to ease.

Looking back, we suspect I'd picked up a virus a couple of weeks earlier when Van had a cold. For him, it was just a mild sniffle. For me, it went straight to my heart. Instead of manifesting as a cold, the virus settled into the membrane around my heart and caused the inflammation. That's motherhood for you – even your toddler's germs can turn into a cardiac emergency.

By Sunday morning, I was stable, but weak. I could only stay on a half dose of the steroids moving forward – any more would endanger the baby. My body was caught between trying to heal and trying to expel the child I was carrying.

My OBGYN returned Monday morning, now 35 weeks and 2 days. "Of course it's you," he said, shaking his head. "Leave it to you to be the first pregnant woman with pericarditis, what a case..."

I was referred to the preterm birth team. They were hoping to get me to 36 weeks for better lung and liver development in the baby. Heidi was fine. But I was fading. My eyes were sunken. I was running on fumes.

Each day, the same cycle: contractions. Valium. Monitoring. Jordan would stop by briefly after work. The verdict was in – I wasn't going home. Not until I had this baby.

On Thursday morning, now 35 weeks and 5 days, the baby started to show signs of distress. My OBGYN came in early and checked the monitors.

"We're not waiting any longer," he said. "Your baby is coming today."

Another C-section was booked for 3:30pm.

I rang Jordan. He had just arrived at work.

"I'm having our baby this afternoon," I said. "It would be nice if you could make it."

Jordan replied, "Oh shit, we really need to start thinking of boys' names." We already had a girl's name sorted, but man – it was tough coming up with another boy's name we loved.

We had nothing. I said, "What about Vincent - Vinnie? Then we'd have Van and Vinnie?"

He left to make arrangements with work. He was rostered to do the ICU rounds that morning. He completed them, had morning tea with a few colleagues, and then made his way to me. That's just who Jordan is. The most reliable person you'll ever meet. He could have easily walked out and said, "My wife's having a baby," and no one would have questioned it. But that would have left the team short – and when you're talking about ICU patients, that matters. I wasn't scheduled until later that afternoon, and it was only 8:30am – plenty of time.

People have said to me since, "How dare he not drop everything and run to your side?" But there was no need. We had a plan. I was safe. He wasn't going to miss the birth. And honestly, it's one of the things I love about him. He doesn't want to put people out. He'll always quietly step in, help where it's needed, and never make a fuss. Van gets that from him – they're so alike.

Back in theatre, hospital policy meant I couldn't watch the procedure. There was a student surgeon assisting this time, alongside my OBGYN. Was I worried? No. Was I stressed? Not at all. I was ready to meet my baby.

But this time, the way the surgical light was positioned, I could just make out the reflection of the surgery in the metal of the overhead lamp. And then – there she was.

A girl.

Thank goodness – we had her name ready.

Heidi. After me. I'm Saara Heidi.

Her full name: Heidi Riitta Elizabeth Jamieson.

Riitta for my mum. Elizabeth for Jordan's.

She was a solid 2.8kg – a good weight for four plus weeks early. I held her for one minute before they whisked her away to the NICU and into a humidicrib. Being early, she needed extra monitoring. Jordan had to head home – Van needed him, and while my parents were helping, we didn't want to burden them. I told him to go. He'd be back the next day.

That night was lonely. I was immobilised from the spinal block – my legs weren't working, Jordan wasn't there, Heidi couldn't come to me, and I couldn't go to her. But as soon as she was out of my body, I started to recover. I wasn't allowed the full steroid dose while breastfeeding but just having her earthside made a difference.

They gave me a photo of her and asked me to hand express colostrum. I rubbed my breasts raw trying to produce every precious drop. I wanted her strong. They fed her through a nasogastric tube using that colostrum. I was determined she'd get the best start possible.

Everyone kept saying, "You'll need to come to terms with going home without her."

My answer was always – "We'll see."

I didn't panic. I wasn't naive. But I knew – we'd go home together.

Heidi beat every milestone.
At 48 hours, she was feeding entirely orally.
At 72 hours, her nasogastric tube was removed.
She was on both breast and bottle, no confusion.

I was never a good milk supplier, no matter how hard I tried. I had to combination feed both of my children. I was just happy that I was able to produce some breast milk.

But I gave it everything.
The routine was relentless:
Breastfeed.
Bottle feed expressed and hand-expressed milk.
Top-up with formula.
Burp.
Settle to sleep.
Machine express.
Hand express.
Sterilise.
Repeat every three hours. I did this for 6 months with Van and 5 months with Heidi.

I tried the teas. The meds. Everything. I just wasn't a high-producing cow – but I was proud to be able to give both my babies a mix of breast and formula, and most importantly – my presence.

The week felt long without Jordan, and I still wasn't allowed to keep Heidi in my room. But each day stretched longer. At three days old, Jordan finally got to hold his daughter.

Other women were struggling with C-section recovery, but I had zero pain. Nothing. Not a flicker. After the pericarditis, my body wasn't registering anything else. I didn't get pain until six weeks later – and then it lasted a month as everything healed.

My paediatrician and the NICU nurses were blown away by Heidi's progress. But still, they pushed for me to go home without her.

I calmly said no.

"If I lose my bed, that's fine. I'll sleep on the couch in the NICU." I'd demonstrated I could safely care for her; she was ready and so was I. "But I'm not going home without my baby."

They extended me one more night.

The next day, the maternity ward was full.

"Okay," I said. "I'll vacate the room. But I'm still not going home without her."

I'd proven I could care for her.

That she was ready.

That I was capable.

And so, I took my daughter home.

We became a family of four.

Looking back now, I realise how tough that week really was. At the time, I was just doing what needed to be done. But it was isolating. Lonely. Nothing like the peaceful, music-filled days we had with Van. With Heidi, it was grit and determination to bring her home.

But once she was in my arms, safe and sound, outside of the hospital – we were whole.

At the time, I didn't think of it as strength. I just thought of it as getting through the week. But looking back, I realise I didn't just advocate for Heidi – I advocated for myself, too. I didn't crumble. I didn't give up. I stayed steady in a situation that nobody had seen before. And I think that's what so many mothers do. Not loudly. Not with fireworks. But with quiet, determined resolve. That's not loud strength. It's lived strength. And it changes everything.

That experience didn't just shape Heidi's entry into the world – it reshaped the way I think about raising girls in it.

Because strength isn't something we tell our daughters they have. It's something they inherit, by watching us live it. Not perform it. It's quiet, practiced, and consistent, the kind they can trust.

Heidi will grow up knowing that bodies can break and rebuild. That you can be vulnerable and still take up space. That you can be scared and still say 'no'.

And that motherhood, like advocacy, like fertility, like founding a company, is often done in rooms where no one is clapping – and yet you do it anyway.

## Putting it into practice

**For our daughters** – Raise daughters who know their worth.

- Model strength with softness:
    - Children absorb what they see far more than what we say. When they see you advocate for your health, stand your ground with grace, and hold space for others, they learn how to do the same.
    - Girls in particular benefit from seeing women model calm strength, especially in high-stress or medical situations.
    - Parental emotional regulation and boundary-setting have long-term impacts on a child's resilience and emotional intelligence (Eisenberg et al., 2005; Kiff et al., 2011).
- Teach assertiveness, not compliance:
    - Move away from rewarding girls only for being 'good' or compliant. Encourage them to voice their opinions, even when they differ.

- - Assertiveness in childhood builds stronger leadership skills and better mental health in adulthood.
  - Girls who are encouraged to voice their opinions show stronger leadership skills and lower risk of internalised stress (Zahn-Waxler et al., 2008).
- Normalise body literacy and rights:
  - Involve daughters in conversations about bodies, health, and reproductive rights from a young age.
  - Share birth stories, talk openly about menstruation, and involve them in decisions where appropriate.
  - Girls who grow up in households with open health dialogue are more likely to report symptoms early, seek help faster, and feel ownership over their wellbeing (Rosenblum & Lewis, 2003; Leaper & Robnett, 2011).

**For parents** – Create an empowering home environment.

- Don't wait for the world to empower her – do it at home:
  - Society may still send mixed signals to your daughter, but your home can be her anchor.
  - Affirm her individuality and strengths consistently, so she develops resilience against external pressures.
  - Maternal stress resilience and warmth can biologically shape a child's long-term stress responses (Yehuda et al., 2016; Grigoriadis et al., 2013).
- Support determination – even when it's hard:
  - Strong-willed daughters may test patience in the short term, but persistence and refusal to give up are the traits that drive change in adulthood.
  - Encourage questioning and critical thinking, even when inconvenient.
  - Longitudinal studies show that strong-willed traits in girls (rule-breaking, questioning authority) are linked to higher income and leadership positions later in life (Miller et al., 2015).

**For all of us** – Because raising girls is everyone's job.

- Model respectful boundaries:
    - Show how to set limits without shame, aggression, or apology.
    - Discipline means teaching, not punishing. Warmth plus structure builds trust and resilience.
    - Consistent boundary-setting and emotional regulation predict stronger emotional intelligence in children (Eisenberg et al., 2005).
- Practise repair, not perfection:
    - Narrate your repair when you lose it ("I was too loud, here's how I want to handle it next time") to model accountability.
    - Letting children see both frustration and repair teaches them what healthy respect looks like.
    - Children of parents who model calm decision-making and repair show stronger self-regulation and coping skills (Kiff et al., 2011).
- Be role models together:
    - Teachers, coaches, uncles, aunties, and community members all influence how girls view themselves.
    - Share stories that celebrate empathy, creativity, and kindness alongside achievement.
    - Exposure to diverse and positive role models improves girls' self-worth and reduces internalised stress (Leaper & Robnett, 2011; Werner & Smith, 2001).

## Behind the chapter: Sources

- Perinatal stress and maternal mental health have profound impacts on bonding, breastfeeding success, and childhood development. When a mother is supported and empowered, even during medical crises, those outcomes improve (Grigoriadis et al., 2013).

- Infant development in NICU environments accelerates with skin-to-skin contact, parental presence, and breastmilk, even partial. Heidi's rapid progress was no accident; the science backs maternal intuition (Conde-Agudelo & Díaz-Rossello, 2016).

- Children of mothers who model self-advocacy and calm decision-making tend to show stronger self-regulation and problem-solving skills (Kiff et al., 2011).

- Girls raised with gender-equitable caregiving and emotionally attuned parenting show higher self-worth and decreased internalised stress, especially when taught to question outdated norms (Leaper & Robnett, 2011).

- Parental emotional regulation and consistent boundary-setting build resilience and emotional intelligence in children, with girls benefiting greatly from calm strength demonstrated in high-stress situations (Eisenberg et al., 2005).

- Encouraging girls to express their opinions, even when they differ from authority, fosters leadership skills and supports better mental health outcomes later in life (Zahn-Waxler et al., 2008).

- Early open dialogue about reproductive health, puberty, and body literacy increases autonomy, self-confidence, and proactive healthcare behaviours in young women (Rosenblum & Lewis, 2003).

- Maternal warmth and resilience have been shown to shape a child's biological stress response, influencing their capacity to cope with challenges well into adulthood (Yehuda et al., 2016).

## THIS SIDE OF THE STORY
## – LETTER TO MY DAUGHTER: MY MISSION, YOUR FIRE

This chapter – and everything that's come before it – isn't just about men's health. It's about shaping a healthier future for all of us, where no one's wellbeing is left out of the conversation.

I started this journey because of a fertility struggle. But what I uncovered was a much bigger truth: that our silence around men's bodies, hormones, and health isn't just harming them – it's harming everyone. Including the women and children who love them. Including the daughters we're raising in the shadows of broken systems.

As I watch my daughter grow up – fiery, curious, loud, and kind – I feel even more urgency around this mission. Because the world she inherits will be shaped by the health and wholeness of the men in it. Her future friendships, partners, leaders, colleagues – all of them – will be shaped by the culture we're building right now, for better or worse. A culture that's long ignored men's pain, shamed their emotions, and turned reproductive health into a 'women's issue'.

But it's not just about changing things for her – it's about what she witnesses in me: how I lead, how I speak up, and what I choose to build.

If I want her to believe she can challenge the status quo, I must show her how it's done. If I want her to use her voice, I need to keep using mine – not perfectly, but honestly and consistently. And that's why this movement was never just about a product.

This movement was never about a product. It was about the people we become when we stop accepting the norm and start asking better questions. It's about raising the bar on what health, strength, masculinity, and legacy really look like.

And the life I lead now? It doesn't look like the one I imagined when I thought motherhood meant slowing down. We never pressed pause – we just rewrote the rules. We take our kids with us. On the hikes. On the adventures. We camp off-grid, cook over open fires, and fall asleep under star-filled skies. It's not always easy, but it's real. It's connected. And it's the kind of life that teaches resilience, wonder, and groundedness. It's not about balancing motherhood and mission – it's about integrating both. Fully. Fiercely. Together.

So, while this started with Cool Beans Underwear®, it will never end there.

Because the ripple effect of one strong voice can reshape a generation.

> My dearest Heidi,
>
> You are fire wrapped in giggles. You are the storm and the stillness.
>
> You came into this world with your own rhythm, and I want you to keep it – especially when others try to change your tune.
>
> You don't have to be easy to love.
>
> Love that's worth anything will rise to meet you.
>
> You don't have to make yourself smaller to be accepted.
>
> The people who matter won't ask you to.
>
> You don't have to be fearless.
>
> You just have to be willing to show up.
>
> This world will tell you a lot about what girls should be. It'll ask you to smile more. Sit quietly. Be agreeable. Don't.
>
> Smile when it's true.
>
> Speak when it matters.
>
> Stand your ground.
>
> You were born from strength.
>
> From hope.

From a fight we almost gave up on.

I want you to see the work I've done, not as sacrifice, but as legacy. A blueprint for what's possible. Not just for men. But for every daughter watching her mum choose purpose over comfort.

This movement – this mission – is for you too.

May you always burn bright. May you always know your worth. May you always trust that your voice was made to be heard.

With all the love I have,
your Mum xxxx

## CHAPTER 19
# SEX, SPERM & SOCIETY

IVF has rightly become a beacon of hope for many families – from same-sex couples and single parents by choice, to those preserving fertility before cancer treatment. Its ability to create families where none could exist before is extraordinary. And yet, even this miracle works best when both partners arrive after optimising their health.

While IVF opens doors, it isn't a cure-all: it works with the eggs and sperm you bring to the clinic. Governments are making it more accessible, subsidising costs to boost populations and offset ageing demographics. But what's often overlooked is that the more we rely on IVF, the more dependent we become on technology to reproduce.

Health must come first, no matter your conception journey. We need to ask: *What can we do before we get to that point, and how can we set ourselves up for the very best outcome?* Medical science offers incredible tools, but the emotional and relational bonds between partners and the health foundations they lay together, remain just as important. IVF works best when it builds on those foundations, not in place of them.

The cultural cost is one that's hard to ignore. When we treat reproduction like a medical procedure, we risk losing sight of its emotional, relational, and biological importance. Even though I never went through IVF, I was more intimate with my OBGYN about scheduling my sex life than with Jordan. In the rush to 'fix' infertility, we risk dehumanising the process. Reproduction becomes something we 'manage' or 'control' through medical means, removing the deep, organic connection that naturally occurs between partners. It also changes the way we view the family unit – turning it into a business transaction, rather than a process of shared love and creation.

Then there's the health cost. IVF is nothing short of extraordinary – a remarkable option that has given countless families hope and children who might never have arrived otherwise. But its success rates are consistently higher when couples take time to optimise health beforehand: nutrition, sleep, stress, environmental exposures, and especially male-factor fertility. IVF works best as a powerful complement to a health-first approach, rather than as a standalone quick fix (which is how many people view IVF – without truly understanding what's involved).

Yet many clinics still don't go deep enough into men's health, sperm quality, or lifestyle factors unless couples know to ask the right questions. It's tempting to skip straight to technology, but doing so can leave the underlying issues unaddressed and the long-term outcome unchanged. What I learned is this: assisted reproduction is an incredible gift, and when paired with simple lifestyle adjustments, open conversations, and thorough medical checks, it gives families the very best chance at a strong and healthy start.

A detailed semen analysis should be every couple's first fertility step, before IVF, before medication. Early insight into sperm DNA integrity and motility can save months of heartache and guide simple lifestyle changes that benefit both natural and assisted conception. Addressing this early can save time, money, and heartache.

In my conversations with females who have gone through multiple rounds of IVF, many have shared that they never once had their partner's sperm analysed. Despite providing sperm samples that were used in IVF procedures, they had no idea about the health of the sperm that was being used. It's a stark reminder of how often male fertility is overlooked in these conversations, and the inherent risk of skipping this critical step in the process. This is one of the biggest gaps in the IVF conversation: male health. Sperm isn't just half the equation – it's half the outcome. Without addressing DNA fragmentation, motility, and morphology early, we're putting every cycle at a disadvantage before it even begins.

Emerging research shows that the environment in which embryos are created – from parental health to lab conditions – can influence long-term health outcomes for children conceived through IVF. While most IVF-conceived children thrive, studies are beginning to explore links between conception conditions and risks for metabolic or cardiovascular differences later in life. This makes pre-IVF health preparation not just about improving the chances of having a child. It's about influencing the lifelong health of that child, from metabolic resilience to emotional wellbeing.

The emotional cost of IVF cannot be overlooked either. No one should underestimate IVF's emotional journey: the injections, the scans, the waiting. By weaving in pre-IVF self-care, stress-reduction practices, and shared coping strategies, you aren't undermining its value; you're building resilience to navigate it with more strength and grace – which can only help IVF outcomes.

For us, the decision was clear: we poured everything into optimising our health naturally. If conception still proved impossible, whether due to sperm integrity or egg quality, I had always wanted to adopt since I was a child, to give a child a home, and so for us, if we couldn't conceive, adoption would be our path. Adoption carries its own journey, but I've always believed that love, not DNA, makes a family. That conviction sits at the heart of my values, yet it's only one of many valid routes to parenthood.

I deeply respect every couple who turns to IVF – its power to create families is nothing short of miraculous. The only misstep is embarking on any path unprepared. Whatever path you choose – natural conception, IVF, surrogacy, donor routes or adoption – remember to lean on the four pillars of fertility, when preparing your health. When IVF enters the conversation, so do schedules, medications, and financial pressures. It's easy for intimacy and emotional connection to get lost in the logistics. Taking intentional time each week to connect outside the fertility conversation, even for a short walk or shared meal, strengthens your resilience for the journey ahead. Nail those basics first, and any medical intervention that follows will have the strongest foundation.

Bringing in a health-first approach doesn't replace IVF – it empowers it. These expert voices remind us that IVF remains a vital, life-changing tool when paired with good prep:

> "IVF remains a safe and effective approach to address fertility issues."
> – Dr Jane Stewart, Chair of the British Fertility Society

> "The report reveals an important truth – infertility does not discriminate. … safe, effective and affordable ways to attain parenthood must be available."
> – Tedros Adhanom Ghebreyesus, WHO Director-General

And from lived experience:

> "With any pregnancy, whether it's through IVF or not, you feel a danger. You have to remain positive and try to relax as much as possible."
> – Céline Dion

IVF has helped countless families conceive. The tension isn't with IVF itself; it's that as treatment has become widely accessible, many of us arrive at the clinic before we've had a chance to work on the basics or even understand what these may be. We need to offer a simple, shared pre-conception plan – for both partners – covering daily stresses, nutrition, exercise and environmental factors, along with semen analysis and maternal checks. Where time allows, build in a short runway of four months of health optimisation while trying naturally; then, if needed, bring IVF in as part of a stronger plan. I understand the urge to move fast when your heart is set on a baby and the clock keeps ticking louder and louder in your head – I've felt this too. What gave me confidence was combining remarkable technology with solid foundations.

In saying all of this, there are many reasons why people should, and will need to, go through IVF, especially those with conditions like endometriosis or blocked seminal ducts where natural conception may be impossible. IVF has provided a pathway to parenthood for many that would otherwise be unattainable. But taking a few months first to address underlying lifestyle and environmental factors before starting treatment can improve outcomes and give your future child the best possible start.

When you're weighing up IVF, it's only natural to wonder about your future child's long-term health, physical strength, emotional resilience or learning potential. Rather than seeing IVF as a 'miracle worker', think of it as a powerful tool that works best when both parents arrive in peak health. Before you book that first cycle, check in on your four pillars of fertility. Each one builds resilience in both partners, improving not just conception chances but the health trajectory of your future child. Just as you wouldn't walk into a marathon untrained, don't walk into IVF without your own pre-game routine. Research shows that factors like sperm DNA integrity and egg quality, both shaped by lifestyle, directly influence embryo development and long-term outcomes. By pairing assisted reproduction with a health-first approach, you honour the science and technology that goes into reproductive services and improve their outcomes. That awareness starts long before IVF – in everyday conversations at home.

Because those early conversations are so often missing, many of us grow up with gaps in understanding that only surface when it matters most. I don't want my children to carry those same blind spots, so I've made openness at home my starting point. And while society hasn't fully caught up with talking about sperm, testes, or menstruation, I've made it a priority to speak openly with my children about their bodies. Even now, while they are still young, I talk to them about my period – when it comes, why I bleed, the use of a menstrual cup, and the importance of managing my menstrual health. If we want a cultural shift in how we approach fertility and health, it starts with what our children see and hear at home. These everyday conversations, whether about menstrual health or protecting sperm quality, sow awareness early, so caring for reproductive health becomes second nature. As Heidi learns menstrual health, Van learns that choices now – nutrition, sleep, and avoiding heat traps like laptops on laps – shape future fertility. These conversations plant seeds early, so caring for reproductive health becomes a part of life, before it's ever urgent.

This isn't just about preparing Heidi for when she starts her own menstrual cycle; it's also about preparing Van. I want him to grow up knowing that respecting and understanding the female body – whether it's his partner's, his friends', or one day, his own child's – is just as important as understanding his own. The conversations we're having now are laying the foundation for the kind of adults they will become – adults who aren't afraid to talk about reproductive health, who aren't embarrassed by the natural processes of their bodies, and who can approach relationships with respect, knowledge, and care.

I've also made it clear that the bathroom door is always open for questions. I want them to see my menstrual cycle for what it is –

nothing to be ashamed of, just a natural part of being human. I want them to know that my body, just like theirs, goes through cycles, changes, and challenges. It's all part of the beautiful process of being human – and something we should celebrate, not hide from. When children grow up seeing fertility and reproductive health as part of everyday life, society itself shifts toward prevention and preparedness.

I can't count how many times I've spoken at events – about sperm, men's testes, their health, and their reproductive responsibility. But each time I do, there's a ripple of discomfort. Grown men squirm in their seats, women and men laugh out loud, and almost every time I speak to someone face-to-face, they will ask, "How do you say all that with a straight face?"

I remember when I was in high school, needing to buy sanitary products while at the shops with a girlfriend. We were there with her mum while she did a grocery shop. My friend leaned in and whispered, as though we were some underage teens, trying to buy alcohol, "Do you want me to ask my mum to buy them for you?" As though the very idea of buying something that my body needed was only for adults and I was doing something that no other girl my age would risk doing for herself. I simply responded, "I'm fine, it's ok."

My friend responded, "Are you sure? It's really no trouble. Are you really going to go in there and buy it yourself?"

This was really the first time that I experienced the sensation that I should be ashamed of my body and what was going on within it. That I need to keep this behind closed doors – to myself. And for a long time after this incident, I did. I didn't speak about my period at school to friends, I kept things to myself. For a long time, I felt embarrassed that this was happening to me – even though I knew it was happening to all my friends and all females. This one encounter – with one friend – was enough for me to feel embarrassed and ashamed of my body, for a normal bodily function.

Now, I talk openly about sperm and testes. Society still hasn't caught up. But what's even more troubling is the way reproduction is increasingly framed as an economic or policy lever – a numbers game to boost birth rates, rather than a deeply personal, human process. Governments pour millions into making IVF cheaper and more accessible, which is a tremendous gift for families who need it. But in doing so, IVF is often positioned as if it were a simple solution to declining fertility rates. Assisted reproduction has revolutionised family building, yet by focusing policy almost exclusively on subsidising technology, we risk overlooking the most powerful intervention of all: improving the everyday health of the individuals involved – especially men. A short-term subsidy may raise birth numbers, but only long-term investment in preventative health will create sustainable fertility for future generations.

Too often, clinical discussions focus solely on egg quality or uterine readiness, but sperm health is just as critical to a successful outcome. Asking your specialist for a detailed semen analysis, diving into factors like DNA fragmentation and motility, and then pairing that insight with simple, evidence-based habits, balanced nutrition, regular exercise, stress management, quality sleep and temperature-regulating underwear, doesn't undermine IVF. It amplifies its potential, ensuring every embryo has the healthiest start possible. In other words, when preparatory health steps become part of your conception plan, you're not sidestepping the technology – you're turbocharging it, enhancing conception outcomes.

IVF can work wonders, but it isn't magic – it can only use the eggs and sperm you bring to the table. All too often, hopeful parents rush straight to the clinic, forgetting that egg and sperm quality influences everything from miscarriage risk to long-term child health. We tend to think inherited mutations are the only danger, overlooking how heat-stressed or chemically burdened sperm introduce spontaneous DNA breaks and epigenetic shifts that ripple through a lifetime. No matter how precise the execution is throughout your reproductive procedure, its impact is limited by what you've already done at home. Fuel your body with wholefoods, clear out toxins, carve out calm, clock solid sleep and keep things cool downstairs, then watch IVF become a true power-up rather than a stand-alone fix.

We're facing a male health crisis right – rising rates of low testosterone, increasing infertility, mental health struggles, and a long-standing neglect of male reproductive health. These issues are deeply interconnected. It's true that, historically, medicine as a whole has often disadvantaged women – from clinical trials designed around male bodies to decades of underfunded research into conditions like endometriosis and menopause. But when it comes to fertility, the pendulum has swung the other way: most attention, treatment and even blame has been directed at women, while men's reproductive health has remained under-examined and under-discussed. It's not about taking focus away from women, but about addressing the imbalance so both partners' health is fully recognised.

It's about empowering people to understand their bodies – all our bodies. Understanding sperm health is just as important as understanding the female reproductive system. If we want to improve natural conception for our children and that of future generations, we need to start with education. We need to shift the narrative that's been so heavily focused on women and move it to a place where both men and women are equally responsible for their reproductive health.

Start by talking openly with your partner about fertility, sperm health, lifestyle choices, and what role both of you play in creating a healthier future. It's not just about checking off medical steps – it's about being active participants in the journey together.

This chapter isn't just about conception. It's about reclaiming ownership of our bodies, our health and our futures. It's about giving men the space to take responsibility for their fertility and wellbeing, just as women have done for generations. And, most importantly, it's about ensuring that the medicalisation of reproduction doesn't overshadow the human reality at its core.

So, let's not rely on technology alone to solve problems that prevention, awareness, and healthier lifestyles could address at their roots. Let's keep asking the harder questions – of ourselves, of our doctors and of our governments. Because the stakes are high: if we only subsidise treatments without investing in health, we risk patching over symptoms rather than solving causes. Prevention and health must sit alongside assisted reproduction, not behind it.

This isn't just a story about sperm – it's about safeguarding the possibility of life itself. By acting now, by widening the conversation and broadening responsibility, we're not only improving our own chances, but shaping a healthier, more fertile future for our children and grandchildren.

## Putting it into practice

**For him** – New, clinic-level actions that most men miss.

- Get a medication and supplement fertility review:
    - Ask your GP or urologist to review your current medications and supplements (e.g., testosterone therapy, anabolic steroids, finasteride/dutasteride, high-dose opioids) and discuss safer alternatives while trying to conceive.
    - Several common drugs suppress what's known as the brain–testis axis, the hormonal pathway where the brain signals the testes to make sperm and testosterone, and this can drop sperm counts to very low levels; planning a switch or pause can help protect fertility.
    - Exogenous testosterone can induce severe oligospermia/azoospermia within months; recovery is typical after cessation but may take 3-12+ months (Endocrine Society CPG; Liu et al., 2017).

- Check testicular health and screen for varicocele:
    - Book a physical exam (and ultrasound if indicated) to assess for varicocele and learn a monthly testicular self-exam routine.
    - Varicoceles are a leading, under-diagnosed cause of impaired semen quality; targeted treatment can improve parameters and natural conception rates.
    - Meta-analyses show varicocele repair improves sperm concentration/motility and increases spontaneous pregnancy rates vs. observation (Baazeem et al., 2011; Marmar, 2007).
- Rule out hidden infections and dental inflammation:
    - Request STI screening (e.g., chlamydia/gonorrhoea) and schedule a dental clean/check for periodontal disease. Treat promptly if positive.
    - Asymptomatic urogenital infections and chronic gum inflammation raise oxidative stress and DNA fragmentation in sperm.
    - Chlamydia-positive semen is linked with higher sperm DNA damage; periodontitis correlates with poorer semen parameters in observational studies (Fertil Steril 2008; J Clin Periodontol 2016).
- Screen for sleep apnea if you snore or wake unrefreshed:
    - If you have loud snoring, witnessed apneas, or daytime sleepiness, ask for a sleep study and treat obstructive sleep apnea (OSA) if present.
    - OSA lowers testosterone and can impair sexual function and metabolic health – treating it helps hormones and energy.
    - Men with OSA show reduced total/free testosterone; treatment (e.g., CPAP, weight loss) improves androgen profile and wellbeing (J Clin Sleep Med 2015 review).

**For her** – High-yield preconception steps rarely covered.

- Check thyroid and iodine status before trying:
  - Ask for TSH, Free T4, ± thyroid antibodies; review iodine intake (iodised salt/prenatal with iodine).
  - Suboptimal thyroid function increases cycle irregularity and miscarriage risk; iodine is essential for thyroid and fetal neurodevelopment.
  - Subclinical hypothyroidism/autoimmunity are associated with impaired fertility and early loss; iodine deficiency remains common in women of reproductive age (ATA Guidelines 2017; WHO).
- Verify immunity and update key vaccinations:
  - Test rubella/varicella immunity and update vaccines (e.g., MMR pre-conception; pertussis/flu per national guidance).
  - Preventable infections can cause severe adverse pregnancy outcomes; confirming immunity before conception is safer than during pregnancy.
  - Preconception immunisation reduces congenital rubella and maternal morbidity; national guidelines recommend checking and updating before pregnancy (Australian Immunisation Handbook/WHO).
- Fast-track a targeted gynae review if you have symptoms:
  - If you experience severe period pain, very heavy bleeding, irregular cycles, acne/hirsutism, or pain with sex, ask for assessment for endometriosis/polycystic ovary syndrome (PCOS) - don't just 'watch and wait'.
  - Early diagnosis and tailored management can improve natural and assisted conception outcomes.
  - Endometriosis and PCOS are major contributors to subfertility; guideline-directed care improves time-to-pregnancy and IVF response (ESHRE/ASRM guidance).

**For us** – Team steps that lift outcomes in and beyond IVF.

- Set a 90-day preconception window – together:
  - Treat the next three months as 'prep time': lock in sleep routines, alcohol limits, and clinic tests for both partners on a shared calendar.
  - Sperm take ~74 days to mature and eggs complete key maturation steps months before ovulation; what you do now shapes gamete quality later.
  - Spermatogenesis ~74 days end-to-end; lifestyle shifts in this window can measurably change semen parameters and cycle quality (Andrology texts; Human Reprod Update reviews).
- Build a joint testing checklist before treatment:
  - Do this as a pair: detailed semen analysis (consider DNA fragmentation if indicated) and male hormones for him; AMH/thyroid ± prolactin for her, plus STI screens for both.
  - Finding issues early prevents wasted cycles and spreads responsibility across both partners.
  - Male factors contribute to ~40-50% of infertility; early, paired evaluation shortens time-to-diagnosis and guides targeted care (ASRM/ESHRE).
- Make an IVF 'informed consent and prep' plan:
  - If IVF is on the table, prepare a question list: lab conditions/quality systems, embryo culture policies, single-embryo transfer, sperm-safe lubricants, and clinic-approved supplements.
  - Clarity up front reduces stress, avoids avoidable risks (e.g., multiples), and aligns your team with best practice.
  - Single-embryo transfer markedly lowers multiple pregnancy risk without reducing cumulative live-birth over successive transfers (ASRM/ESHRE guidance).

## Behind the chapter: Sources

- Lifestyle choices have a measurable impact on sperm health. Diet, alcohol consumption, smoking, environmental toxins, and stress can significantly affect sperm quality. Adopting proper nutrition, regular exercise, and stress management can improve sperm count, motility, and overall fertility (Agarwal et al., 2014).

- Environmental pollutants are directly linked to reduced male fertility. Chemicals found in plastics, pesticides, and industrial pollutants can impair sperm count and reproductive function, contributing to long-term fertility decline (Sharpe, 2010).

- Male fertility is declining at a global scale. Sperm counts in Western men have dropped by more than 50% over the past 40 years, indicating an urgent need to address male reproductive health alongside female fertility (Levine et al., 2017).

- IVF carries emotional and psychological costs. The stress, isolation, and anxiety associated with IVF are well documented, with many couples reporting feelings of emotional exhaustion during treatment. This highlights the need for better mental health support throughout fertility journeys (Wischmann et al., 2009).

- Advances in IVF raise new ethical considerations. The increasing ability to select embryos for health or physical traits has sparked debates about genetic selection and the potential risks of eugenics (Baker, 2006).

- Poor sperm quality remains an overlooked contributor to infertility. While IVF is a critical tool for conception, it does not address the root causes of male infertility, with sperm quality – not just quantity – playing a decisive role in reproductive success (Zohni et al., 2014).

# PART V
## A NEW KIND OF STRENGTH

**CoolBeans**

# CHAPTER 20
# THE FUTURE WE'RE BUILDING

My mother always told me that I was her 'miracle baby'. That I was destined for great things. For the longest time, I didn't fully understand the weight of that phrase. Her belief wasn't unfounded – it came from the sheer improbability of my existence, a story that shaped not just my childhood but the way I see my purpose today.

My mum's journey to have me wasn't conventional. After losing her third son, she had her fallopian tube tied to her only functioning ovary, thinking she would never conceive again. At 41, she thought she was dying or had cancer – but discovered that in fact she was three months pregnant with me. Her non-functional ovary – one doctors said had never and would never work – suddenly released an egg. The doctors were shocked, and when Mum went to the hospital to give birth, the nurses told her it was impossible to have a daughter. They had already delivered 5 girls that day, and the idea of a 6th girl was inconceivable. Mum had to have an emergency C-section, and when she awoke from the anaesthetic, the nurse brought me to her and said, "We have wonderful news for you, you had a little girl. We knew you wanted a daughter, and we didn't think it was possible, but here you are."

And Mum just began to cry and cry as she held me.

Mum had always wanted a daughter and had already chosen my name – Saara Heidi Johanna – back when she was pregnant with my eldest brother. When she first held me, defying all medical odds, she called me her 'miracle baby'. It was in that moment that she knew, without a doubt, that I was meant for something extraordinary. I didn't feel extraordinary growing up. I struggled at school and didn't excel in any particular area. But Mum always saw something in me, something I couldn't see in myself. Her belief in me was unwavering, and it became the foundation of everything I've done. Maybe, just maybe, that one egg from a broken ovary was released to bring me here to this point – to do this. And now, looking at what I've built, I believe it too.

Growing up with that sense of destiny, that belief that I was meant for something bigger, shaped my perspective. It wasn't just about proving my worth to my mother – it was about believing in the importance of my journey, my health, and the choices I made. And as I began to build Cool Beans, I realised how much our society needed a change. We needed to address reproductive health for everyone, and I knew that to make an impact, we had to open the conversation, breaking down barriers, and encouraging men to take control of their health. It wasn't just about fertility – it was about creating a space for men to take responsibility for their bodies, for their lives, and for their future.

When I started Cool Beans, it wasn't just about fertility or infertility; it was about reimagining how we think about reproductive health for people of all genders. But much like the foundation my mother laid for me, a big part of that mission was giving my children the same opportunities I had in terms of education. For a long time, Jordan and I had to scrape together what we could: developing Cool Beans Underwear® and, when the time came, private schooling too. We were determined to send our kids to the same private school I attended. There's something grounding about seeing them walk those same halls, about providing them with the opportunities that, while challenging, has now become part of the legacy we're building for them.

The recognition Cool Beans has received over the past year, from the *Today* show to podcast appearances, has been nothing short of amazing, but also humbling. It's incredible to see how many people are now joining the conversation about men's health – about fertility, testosterone, and the larger issues that have been swept under the rug for far too long. Cool Beans isn't just a product – it's a reflection of the movement we're helping to lead. As we shine a light on male reproductive health, we're also sparking a shift in how society views men's well-being.

But none of this would have been possible without the unwavering support of partners like testhim™ in the UK, who became our first distributor, advancing reproductive health for all, breaking barriers and driving change where it's sorely needed. testhim's efforts in raising awareness about men's fertility and ensuring that men's health is not overlooked in the larger conversation about reproduction are just the beginning. Together, we're rewriting the narrative. But our work doesn't stop with men's health alone; it's about holistically addressing fertility and reproduction, ensuring we don't bypass the deep-rooted issues that lead to infertility in the first place.

We're witnessing a growing societal shift, albeit slowly. We see more and more advocates for preventative health, but society is still primarily reactive when it comes to healthcare. We treat the symptoms of infertility with IVF and other interventions, but rarely do we address the core issue – the declining fertility and reproductive health that's impacting both men and women. Our medical systems, our societal approach, still focus on treating problems once they've already manifested, rather than investing in prevention. And this, my friends, is a huge part of why we're facing a crisis in men's reproductive health. We're playing catch-up, rather than taking proactive measures to safeguard future generations.

This is why Cool Beans matters so much. While IVF can be transformative for many, it shines brightest when preceded by proactive, holistic reproductive health for everyone. If we can shift the narrative towards proactive care, we can start addressing the root causes of fertility struggles rather than just the symptoms. And that shift is not just important for men's reproductive health – it's crucial for the future of natural conception itself, for our children and their children.

> "We can say with a high degree of confidence that there have been at least 12 million IVF babies since the world's first in 1978."
> - David Adamson, Chair of ICMART

When we officially launched Cool Beans Underwear®, I thought things would get easier. I'd put in years of work, countless sleepless nights, and immense sacrifices to get to this point. I thought the hardest part was behind me. But the truth is, without a team, and with the constant pressure to grow the brand, enhance our impact, write a book, and tackle new challenges, my workload increased.

I've learned that launching isn't the end of the journey – it's just the beginning. The pressure to do more, to reach more people, to make a bigger impact, can feel overwhelming at times. But here's the thing – I wouldn't change it for the world. The more I see our impact on individuals, families, and the broader reproductive-health conversation, the more I know it's all worth it. We're not just changing men's health – we're also changing the future for our kids.

Watching Van now planning his own business, I'm excited to see where he takes it, as it's a great idea. Seeing Heidi support him, helping around the house, and wanting to contribute, fills me with pride. I see the determination and drive in them, and I know that Cool Beans isn't just changing the conversation for this and the next generation, but for the right now, in this house, for these kids. I'm proud of what we've built,

## The future we're building

and I'm excited for what the future holds, even if it means working harder than ever.

But that hard work will not produce results if we don't start to understand how our health is being impacted. We are living very different lives today than we were 50 years ago. Our environment, our diets, our increasingly sedentary lifestyles – they're all playing a significant role in the decline of fertility. Excess testicular heat, the accumulation of chemicals and toxins in the environment, microplastics in our food, and nutrient-poor diets are all compounding factors in the erosion of men's health. The truth is, the biological clock is ticking faster than most realise, and the consequences of inaction are significant.

Men today have lower sperm counts than their fathers and grandfathers did. Testosterone levels are declining year on year, and we're seeing higher rates of infertility. We're having more children suffering with mental health, and with mental and physical disabilities than ever before. The very changes in the way we live – our diet, our environment, our lack of movement – are directly affecting our biological health. The most concerning part? Testosterone levels aren't just affecting fertility; they are linked to nearly every aspect of men's health. Lower testosterone affects muscle mass, bone density, energy levels, mental clarity, and mood. It impacts men's ability to function in every facet of their lives, from work to relationships.

But here's the kicker: taking artificial testosterone doesn't just solve the problem; it makes it worse. When men go on testosterone replacement therapy (TRT), they stop producing their own testosterone, but they also stop producing sperm. So, while you might feel better, you are also making it even harder, potentially impossible, to have kids naturally or with your own sperm.

The truth is, taking artificial testosterone messes with a lot more than just fertility. It can affect your muscle mass, your energy, your mood, and even your heart health. It's a solution that masks the real problem – and often delays the lifestyle changes that would improve health naturally. Plus, it can create a cycle where you depend more and more on testosterone supplementation; while individual symptoms may improve, overall health and longevity likely won't be improved, and it also affects production of your other hormones.

It's important to understand that fixing testosterone with supplements won't fix the underlying issues, like lifestyle or stress. Focusing on those first, with healthy habits and balanced living, is a much better way to go if you want long-term results.

This is why I'm so passionate about what we're doing. Our work isn't about a single product; it's about shifting how men's health is approached. If we can improve testosterone levels naturally, we can improve every aspect of men's health. We can protect fertility, mental health, physical health, and wellbeing, and in doing so, we can create a healthier future for the next generation.

For myself, struggling with infertility wasn't just about wanting to have a child – it was about understanding the deeper, underlying issues that were affecting us. Jordan and I faced infertility for years. The toll it took on us wasn't just emotional – it was a physical and mental battle that we both had to face head-on. But as we worked through it, it became clear that the problem wasn't just infertility – it was about men's health in general. The lack of focus on men's reproductive health, the silence around it, was what fuelled my determination to keep pushing forward. It wasn't just about conceiving; it was about understanding the broader picture – how men's health, particularly their reproductive health, had been ignored for far too long.

The root causes of infertility were often linked to broader health issues: diet, stress, environmental factors, and lifestyle choices all played a huge part in male fertility. And as I dug deeper, it became clear: this wasn't just about us. It was about men everywhere. Men weren't being educated about their own bodies, about how their health directly impacted their ability to reproduce.

That's when Cool Beans came into the picture. It wasn't just about fertility – it became about men's health overall. The mission shifted from trying to get pregnant to addressing the underlying health issues that were affecting men's reproduction, testosterone levels, mental health, and physical wellbeing. It's about giving men the tools to understand their own health and take control, not just when they're trying to have children, but in every part of their lives.

The future of natural conception isn't just a dream – it's a tangible goal. It's a future where we take control of our health, starting today. It's about empowering men to own their health, to make decisions that will improve not only their fertility but their overall wellbeing. And it's about building a culture of care, not just for us, but for the generations to come. The change we need won't come from a pill, a treatment, AI or artificial wombs – it will come from informed choices, daily action, and a collective will to protect our health before it's too late. It's time to act. To prevent. To protect. To shape our children's future, together.

## Putting it into practice

**For him** – Holistic health beyond reproductive focus.

- Practice mindful movement:
    - Integrate mindfulness into your movement practices, such as walking, stretching, or yoga. These activities not only reduce stress but help you reconnect with your body and promote overall health.
    - Mindful movement helps decrease cortisol levels, improve circulation, and support your body's natural functions. Regular physical activity is crucial for both mental and physical wellbeing.
    - Studies show that mindfulness-based activities can reduce stress and improve physical health by balancing hormones like

cortisol, which impacts both fertility and overall health (Zeidan et al., 2010).

- Prioritise sleep hygiene:
    - Commit to a consistent sleep routine. Aim for at least 7–8 hours of quality sleep every night. Avoid excessive screen time before bed and aim for a calming evening routine to enhance sleep quality.
    - Poor sleep has been linked to reduced testosterone levels and increased stress, both of which negatively affect health and fertility. Quality sleep supports hormone regulation, including testosterone.
    - Research shows that sleep deprivation can reduce testosterone levels by up to 15%, affecting fertility and overall wellbeing (Dawson et al., 2014).

**For her** – Take care of your overall wellbeing.

- Create a stress-relief ritual:
    - Build a daily stress-relief ritual that can include activities like meditation, stretching, or enjoying a quiet evening routine. Consistency is key.
    - Chronic stress is one of the biggest disruptors of hormonal balance, which affects reproductive health and overall wellbeing. Taking time for yourself each day can make a significant difference to your hormonal health.
    - Studies indicate that mindfulness and relaxation exercises, such as meditation, can significantly lower cortisol levels, improving hormonal balance and mental health (Zadeh et al., 2015).
- Eat the rainbow:
    - Aim to eat a variety of colourful vegetables and fruits daily. Each colour provides different nutrients and antioxidants essential for your body's natural functions.

- A diverse diet packed with antioxidants, vitamins, and minerals helps reduce oxidative stress and supports overall health, including reproductive health. A well-rounded diet can improve egg health and menstrual cycle regularity.
- Research highlights that eating a variety of nutrient-dense foods, particularly colourful fruits and vegetables, enhances reproductive health by providing essential antioxidants that protect eggs from oxidative damage (Hassan et al., 2013).

**For us** – Strengthen emotional and physical health together.

- Commit to mutual health goals:
  - Set shared health goals, whether it's cooking healthier meals together or taking evening walks. Make these goals fun and engaging to strengthen your emotional and physical connection.
  - Working together on health goals fosters teamwork, accountability, and a deeper connection. It also benefits both partners' overall health and can improve your fertility journey.
  - Families and partners who engage in shared health initiatives, such as improving diet or exercise, have been shown to have improved fertility outcomes and better emotional wellbeing (Agarwal et al., 2014).
- Practice open communication about health:
  - Have regular check-ins about your physical and emotional health. Share not only challenges but also wins and improvements. Transparency strengthens intimacy and reduces stress.
  - Open communication helps reduce feelings of isolation, fosters understanding, and builds trust. Regular check-ins about health can decrease emotional stress, which positively impacts fertility and wellbeing.
  - Research from the American Psychological Association found that couples who engage in open health discussions experience improved mental health and greater emotional support during fertility struggles (APA, 2018).

## Behind the chapter: Sources

- Men's sperm counts have declined significantly over the past few decades. Studies show a marked decrease in sperm count in Western men, linked to environmental and lifestyle factors such as exposure to toxins, poor diet, and sedentary living. This decline has significant implications for fertility and overall health (Levine et al., 2017).

- Testicular heat is a major factor in reduced sperm production. Prolonged exposure to heat – often from tight clothing, prolonged sitting, or sedentary lifestyles – can damage sperm quality and lead to a decline in fertility. The optimal temperature for sperm production is a few degrees below body temperature, and anything that raises testicular heat can negatively impact production (Koskelo et al., 2005).

- Poor diet and nutrient deficiencies contribute to infertility in men. A diet rich in antioxidants, omega-3 fatty acids, and zinc can improve sperm health and motility. Research shows that men with poor diets are more likely to have lower sperm quality and count, and a balanced diet is crucial for improving reproductive health (Agarwal et al., 2014; Hassan et al., 2013).

- Artificial testosterone therapy suppresses natural testosterone production and can lead to infertility. Men who undergo testosterone replacement therapy (TRT) often experience a decrease in sperm production, as the body stops producing its own testosterone. This can make it harder to conceive naturally and creates a reliance on external testosterone (Zohni et al., 2014).

- Sleep quality has a direct impact on male hormone health. Sleep deprivation can reduce testosterone levels by up to 15%, affecting fertility, mood, and overall wellbeing (Dawson et al., 2014).

- Stress management is critical for both partners in a fertility journey. Chronic stress elevates cortisol levels, which can disrupt hormonal balance in men and women. Mindfulness-based activities have been shown to reduce cortisol and improve physical health (Zeidan et al., 2010; Zadeh et al., 2015).

- IVF is a solution for many, but it does not address the root causes of infertility. While IVF has helped many couples conceive, it bypasses the natural process of reproduction and does not solve underlying health issues such as poor sperm quality or lifestyle factors. Addressing these issues before resorting to IVF can improve long-term reproductive health (Sharma et al., 2018).

- Testosterone levels are declining globally. The decline in testosterone levels in men is linked to lifestyle factors, including stress, poor diet, and environmental toxins. Low testosterone affects not just fertility but also muscle mass, bone density, mood, energy levels, and overall wellbeing (Travison et al., 2007).

## THIS SIDE OF THE STORY
### – THE RIPPLE EFFECT

There are moments – still – where I look at what we've built and think, how did we get here?

Orders are coming in from all over the world. Clinicians are recommending Cool Beans to their patients. We've been on national television, featured in articles I once dreamed of, invited onto podcasts I've followed for years. And somehow, I've found myself a finalist for Innovator of the Year, Disruptor of the Year, and awarded for Social Enterprise Excellence for helping couples conceive healthier children.

It blows me away.

This all started because we wanted a baby. We were desperate for answers – and when none came, we went looking ourselves. I never imagined that search would become a business, a movement, or a mission that would touch so many lives.

There have been so many points I wanted to give up. When everything in life and business collided and felt so impossibly heavy. But then I'd get a message from a couple who conceived. Or a note from someone recovering after cancer surgery. Or a clinician reaching out to say, "This changes everything." And I'd remember: this was never just underwear.

We've done something that no one else has done. Scientists have been trying to solve testicular heat and reproductive decline for over 50 years – and somehow, we did it. Just the two of us. A husband-and-wife team. No corporate machine. No big funding behind us. Just a belief that this mattered, and the sheer, exhausting persistence to see it through.

And we didn't just make something that works – we made something men actually want to wear. Support without discomfort. A custom fit for real bodies. No more readjusting, no more tight compression, no more awkward seams. We solved a problem most people didn't even realise was affecting their health, their hormones, and their future.

That's the part that gets me most. This tiny thing – a change in underwear – is reshaping conversations in bedrooms, clinics, and living rooms around the world. Men are feeling seen. Couples are feeling hopeful. Families are being built. Not just physically, but emotionally too.

This isn't just underwear. It's agency. It's action. It's a shift in how we talk about health – not just for men, but for everyone who loves them.

And here's what I know for sure: the ripple effect is real.

This idea – this product – has become so much more. It's a quiet rebellion against complacency. A challenge to the way things have always been done. And it's proof that change doesn't have to start big. It can start with one family. One couple. One determined woman with a vision, a baby on her hip, and no backup plan.

Now, that ripple is becoming a wave and we're not done yet.

**CoolBeans**

# CHAPTER 21
# FUTUREPROOFING MANHOOD

We may be the last generation to take natural conception for granted. I didn't start Cool Beans to change the world – yet here, watching Van throw crusts to the chickens and Heidi shriek at the butcherbird, I realise I'm building a future they deserve – that they can thrive in. One where they have the option to conceive naturally and live long, strong, vibrant lives – and not inherit the slow, silent crisis we're failing to confront. If we don't make changes today, the future for our children will be in peril.

Without venture capital financial backing, but with family support, a purpose, and a child in my arms who had become my entire life, I knew exactly what I needed to do – everything in my power to secure a healthier future for my kids. That clarity gave me the courage to keep going. Cool Beans wasn't born in a lab. It was built in late nights, raw conversations, sacrifice, and relentless belief. And now, it's part of something bigger: a movement to redefine what men's health looks like in the modern world.

As a bioscience student, I learned that even a 1°C rise in a bull's scrotal heat devastates sperm quality. It was textbook knowledge in

Northern Australia – bulls in northern Queensland were often less fertile during warmer times of the year and heatwaves, and you wouldn't take sperm straws for artificial insemination in those conditions. Yet no one ever applied this insight to men. That omission stuck with me for years, and when I came back to it while building Cool Beans, I couldn't unsee it. The science had been there all along – we just hadn't applied it to humans.

Today, as global temperatures rise, so does this risk. Cities are hotter. Commutes are longer. Our lifestyles are more sedentary. And yet, men are still told nothing about the role heat plays in their health. It's time we changed that.

Right now, we're living in a time where more organisations are rising up, to support men's mental health, reproductive health, fitness, and disease management. But most of them are operating in silos – addressing individual issues, one at a time. What's still missing is a connected view. One that recognises that these challenges are symptoms of a larger pattern. A deeper shift in the male body, shaped by how we live now.

We're seeing a global trend of falling testosterone – estimated to be declining by roughly 1% each year. That may not sound like much until you realise that Testosterone acts like a master switch for men's health. It affects everything from energy and motivation to bone density, heart health, libido, fertility, and emotional resilience. When it drops, it doesn't just impact sex drive – it impacts the entire trajectory of a man's life.

But testosterone decline isn't happening in a vacuum. It's driven by modern life itself: more sedentary routines, processed food, exposure to endocrine-disrupting chemicals, and a growing detachment from body awareness. All of these physical shifts are reinforced by culture – by the way we live, work, eat, and even talk (or don't talk) about men's health. And that's why futureproofing manhood isn't just about health

– it's about culture. It's about the stories we tell our sons. The habits we pass down. The silent assumptions we leave unchallenged.

To shift the future, we need a two-pronged approach. Biology responds to environment, and behaviour reshapes both. When daily life nudges heat, sleep, diet and stress in the wrong direction, hormones follow – and so do energy, mood and fertility.

First, we need to help today's men understand what's happening to their biology. That their health isn't failing because they're weak – but because the world they live in wasn't built with their long-term wellbeing in mind. Once we name the problem, we can change it. We can educate men on how testicular heat, stress, diet, and toxins all affect testosterone and fertility. We can provide tools – not shame – to help them make empowered choices.

Second, we need to prepare the next generation to navigate a changing health landscape, from understanding how lifestyle influences fertility and hormones to recognising early warning signs that call for preventative care. Tomorrow's strength will rest on being informed, proactive, and emotionally agile. We must teach boys that real resilience includes vulnerability, that masculinity thrives on self-awareness, and that asking for help is a mark of leadership, not weakness. Equip them with these skills, and we don't just improve their chances of thriving, we reshape the future of men's health.

Just the other day, I watched Van and Heidi eat their sandwiches out the back. The dog raced the chickens for fallen crusts. A butcherbird swooped in and beat them all. It made me reflect on the circle of life we see play out daily on our little farm – from chicks hatching to old hens nearing the end. I've taught my kids about that cycle. About life and death. About the importance of what we put in our bodies today to shape our future health. But lately, I've started asking: what kind of circle of life will they inherit? Will natural conception still be an option? Will their generation struggle with rising rates of depression, autoimmune issues, infertility?

There were so many moments I questioned everything. When the prototypes didn't work. When money ran out. When the quiet voice in my head whispered, "What if this doesn't matter?" But then I'd get an email – from a couple who'd almost given up who were now expecting, or a man who no longer feared chronic pain. Each message was a reminder that this wasn't just about a product – it was about rewriting someone's future. It was about giving people hope in a world that keeps taking it away.

The truth is that this work is exhausting. There's no big team. No investor millions. Just me, my husband, a product born of desperation, and a mission that keeps getting louder. I answer messages at midnight. I ship orders with kids in the car. I cry some days. But I keep going – because stopping now would mean handing the next generation a problem we could have fixed. Because the cost of doing nothing is too great.

The answer depends on what we do now. On whether we take this moment seriously. Whether we act with urgency, compassion, and clarity. Cool Beans is one part of the solution – but this mission goes beyond one product. It's about rebuilding the very foundation of men's health – and in doing so, protecting families, communities, and generations to come.

We may be the last generation to take natural conception for granted – and I'm not okay with that. If I can do something about it, I will. That's the entire point of this work.

I challenge you to share one insight from this chapter with a father, coach, or teacher today. Conversations spark awareness, and awareness drives change – and change is how we protect the next generation's ability to conceive, connect, and live well.

## Mini Q&A – What people still want to know

**Q: Does underwear really make a difference?**
A: Yes – if it's designed with male anatomy in mind. Traditional styles often trap heat and offer poor scrotal support. Cool Beans Underwear® uses an external anatomical pouch to promote airflow and reduce heat – a key factor in supporting sperm health, testosterone, and comfort. While we can't make direct medical claims, it's built to address risk factors backed by science.

**Q: Is sperm health really linked to overall health?**
A: Absolutely. Sperm is a sensitive health marker, reflecting things like oxidative stress, inflammation, hormone balance, and even sleep quality. If sperm health declines, it's often an early warning sign that other body systems may also be under pressure.

**Q: Why haven't I heard this before?**
A: Because men's fertility has rarely been prioritised – socially or clinically. Historically, the focus has been on women, and only recently has research revealed how crucial men's preconception health is for both fertility and the long-term health of future generations.

**Q: What's the first step to improve hormone health?**
A: Start small with proven habits: reduce testicular heat, get consistent good-quality sleep, move your body daily, and keep alcohol and ultra-processed foods in check. These simple steps have compounding benefits over time.

**Q: How can I get my testosterone tested – and what levels are optimal?**
A: Your GP can order a blood test, ideally early in the morning when levels peak. Two main measures are worth knowing:

- Total testosterone – overall amount in your blood.
- Free testosterone – the biologically active portion.

You'll see testosterone reported in either:

- nmol/L – nanomoles per litre (used in Australia, UK, and most of the world).
- ng/dL – nanograms per decilitre (used mainly in the USA).

Here's a general guide for *total testosterone*:

| Age Range | Avg. Range (nmol/L) | Optimal Range (nmol/L) | Avg. Range (ng/dL) | Optimal Range (ng/dL) |
|---|---|---|---|---|
| 20–29 years | 21–30 | 25–30 | 606–865 | 715–865 |
| 30–39 years | 18–27 | 22–27 | 519–779 | 634–779 |
| 40–49 years | 15–25 | 20–25 | 432–721 | 577–721 |
| 50+ years | 12–22 | 17–22 | 346–634 | 491–634 |

If you're near the lower end and feeling fatigued, unfocused, low in libido, or emotionally flat, it's worth further testing (free testosterone, LH, SHBG) before jumping to medication – lifestyle changes can often make a real difference.

**Q: What can I do if my partner won't listen?**
A: Lead with empathy, not pressure. Resistance often comes from fear, shame, or feeling overwhelmed. Suggest learning together – share a short article, watch a quick video, or open a casual conversation. This is about shared hope, not blame.

**Q: What about exercise, alcohol, diet, and medication?**
A: All of these matter. Overtraining can lower testosterone. Alcohol and processed food impact gut, liver, and hormone health. Certain

medications can affect sperm production. You don't need to be perfect – just aware. Always consult your doctor before changing any prescribed treatment.

## Putting it into practice

### Youth: For him

- Cool the core – limit long hours of seated screen time:
    - Encourage boys to take movement breaks every 30–60 minutes when gaming or studying. Ideally, have them stand or stretch between sessions.
    - Long sitting sessions increase scrotal heat, which can suppress testosterone production and impair sperm development.
    - Just 20 minutes of sitting can raise scrotal heat by up to 2.2°C – enough to suppress testosterone and sperm production (Koskelo et al., 2005).
- Reduce ultra-processed foods:
    - Limit intake of fast food, soft drinks, and processed snacks. Replace with whole foods like eggs, fruit, oats, and lean proteins.
    - Diets high in ultra-processed foods reduce testosterone and increase oxidative stress – harming hormonal balance and long-term health.
    - Men who consumed more than 50% of calories from processed foods had significantly lower testosterone levels (Hall et al., 2019).

### Youth: For her

- Track symptoms early:
    - Encourage teens to use a cycle tracking app to note pain, mood, flow, and irregularities – not just when their period arrives.

- Early tracking helps identify PCOS or endometriosis symptoms and empowers girls to understand their own hormonal rhythms.
  - Early intervention in adolescent PCOS symptoms can improve outcomes and reduce future infertility risk (Teede et al., 2010).
- Cut down plastics and endocrine disruptors:
  - Avoid heating or storing food in plastic containers. Use glass or stainless steel alternatives, especially for warm meals and drinks.
  - Plastics (especially BPA and phthalates) can interfere with oestrogen and progesterone balance during puberty and reproductive development.
  - Understanding her cycle from an early age not only supports her own reproductive health, but also contributes to stronger couple fertility outcomes in adulthood – where both partners' health plays an equal role in conception.
  - BPA exposure is linked to earlier puberty onset and increased menstrual irregularity in teenage girls (Harley et al., 2011).

**For parents**

- Start the body literacy conversations early:
  - Create safe, shame-free moments to talk about bodies – during drives, around the dinner table, or casually during daily life.
  - Normalising body talk makes it easier for kids to ask questions later, including about fertility, puberty, and sexual health.
  - Teens who feel comfortable discussing health with parents report fewer risky behaviours and better long-term wellbeing (Widman et al., 2016).
- Teach the link between daily habits and future health:
  - Use examples like a daily walk or dental hygiene to illustrate how small daily actions lead to future outcomes. Then extend this to hormones, sleep, and food.
  - When kids understand that health is compounding – not reactive – they're more likely to build sustainable habits. This

includes recognising how everyday actions affect hormone balance, fertility potential, and long-term wellbeing.
- Health behaviours adopted in adolescence strongly predict adult disease risk and fertility outcomes (Sawyer et al., 2012).

## Behind the chapter: Sources

- Sperm production and testosterone synthesis require the testes to be 2–4°C cooler than core body temperature. Prolonged heat from tight underwear, polyester fabrics, prolonged sitting, or warm environments can significantly reduce both sperm count and hormone output (Mieusset & Bujan, 1995; Shafik, 1992).

- Sitting for just 20 minutes can raise scrotal heat by up to 2.2°C – enough to impair testosterone production and suppress sperm development (Koskelo et al., 2005).

- Polyester underwear generates static and traps heat, which has been shown to significantly reduce sperm count and motility (Shafik, 1992).

- Sperm quality is closely linked to systemic health, including oxidative stress, inflammation, endocrine disruption, sleep quality, and metabolic function. Declines in sperm quality often indicate broader health challenges (Agarwal et al., 2014).

- Despite contributing to 50% of infertility cases, male factors are routinely under-evaluated. Many clinics fail to assess DNA fragmentation, oxidative stress markers, or subtle hormone imbalances – especially when female conditions like PCOS or endometriosis are present (Esteves et al., 2012).

- Assisted reproduction still relies on the foundational quality of sperm and egg. Poor sperm DNA integrity can affect embryo development, implantation success, and miscarriage risk – even with IVF or Intracytoplasmic Sperm Injection (ICSI) (Simon et al., 2017).

- Studies show that average testosterone levels have dropped by approximately 1% per year over the past few decades. This has serious implications for male energy, cognition, fertility, muscle mass, cardiovascular health, and mood (Travison et al., 2007).
- Diets high in ultra-processed foods are linked to lower testosterone and increased oxidative stress, negatively impacting hormonal balance (Hall et al., 2019).
- Paternal age and health at conception influence not just sperm quality but also offspring's long-term outcomes – including risks for neurodevelopmental disorders, metabolic conditions, and even shorter telomeres in children (Kovac et al., 2013; Sharma et al., 2015).
- BPA exposure during adolescence is associated with earlier onset of puberty and increased menstrual irregularities (Harley et al., 2011).
- Early identification and management of adolescent PCOS symptoms can improve long-term reproductive outcomes and reduce infertility risk (Teede et al., 2010).
- Adolescents who feel comfortable discussing sexual health with parents engage in fewer risky behaviours and report better long-term wellbeing (Widman et al., 2016).
- Health behaviours established in adolescence strongly predict adult disease risk, hormone balance, and fertility outcomes (Sawyer et al., 2012).
- Emerging research shows that paternal postnatal depression is linked to higher risk of emotional, behavioural, and social difficulties in children. These issues may originate before birth and go unrecognised until the postpartum period (Ramchandani et al., 2008).

- Total testosterone doesn't always reflect what's biologically active. Free testosterone – the unbound fraction – is responsible for regulating libido, muscle growth, energy levels, and mood. Assessing both total and free testosterone offers a clearer picture of male hormonal health (Wu et al., 2008).

**CoolBeans**

## CHAPTER 22
## GLOBAL BLIND SPOTS

We realised we'd stumbled onto a global blind spot in men's reproductive care – the lack of tools, language, and clinical focus on male fertility – the day our first order arrived from Dubai. A handful of initial enquiries grew into messages from clinicians in Denmark, distributors in the UK, and patients from every continent. Each one crying out for an entry point into a conversation no one else was starting – a conversation that, until now, had no clear beginning. Curious questions from clinicians who said they'd never had a tangible way to start conversations with male patients. That's when I realised: the need wasn't just local – it was global, understood by people everywhere who were already seeking answers, and just needed someone to articulate the problem and offer a path forward.

I remember standing at the clothesline, reading a message from a doctor in Kuwait who had just prescribed Cool Beans to a patient recovering from cancer. I had to read it twice. Not because I didn't believe him – but because part of me still couldn't believe we'd built something that could help a man halfway across the world. No venture capital. No manufacturing background – just a medical researcher with a passion and a purpose, and with the fight to prove it mattered.

Each message revealed unique challenges. For example, in the Middle East, clinicians explained how cultural taboos often made it difficult to discuss reproductive health with male patients. But having a real, physical product in hand gave them a neutral, non-threatening entry point – a way to shift the conversation from awkward to approachable and finally begin breaking through the silence.

In Scandinavia, where preventative frameworks are well developed and health education begins early, there's a strong focus on public health – yet male reproductive health still falls behind. Sperm testing is often delayed until after female-focused interventions have failed, and hormonal testing for men remains rare. However, some countries like Norway and Finland are exploring more balanced approaches, with pilot programs introducing early education about fertility for both sexes. It's progress – slow, but promising.

In the UK, more attention is being given to male fertility and reproductive health. Initiatives like testhim™ are paving the way, offering sperm testing kits, raising public awareness, and creating online tools to educate and support men before they even begin trying to conceive. It's a model that doesn't just respond to crisis – it aims to prevent it. While the broader system still tends to focus on women first, these initiatives show how we can begin to shift the norm. But without systemic policy changes and equal diagnostic pathways for men, these efforts risk becoming isolated wins instead of nationwide progress.

In Australia, people are becoming more vocal about men's health, particularly in the farming and regional communities where male suicide rates have been tragically high. These conversations are gaining traction through mental health campaigns, but we still struggle to connect the dots between reproductive, mental, and physical health. When I speak to clinicians here, they often tell me that unless a man is actively trying to conceive, no one is looking at his hormone health at all.

Imagine if every GP appointment included a two-second testicular health check. Or if school health classes taught simple heat management and hormone basics alongside biology. Small, local changes ripple into global progress.

I've also seen the contrast first-hand. Back in 2010, I lived in South Africa during a gap year where I trained and worked as a Big Five animal field guide. It was the best year of my life – tracking wildlife, teaching tourists about ecosystems, and feeling completely connected to nature. But it also revealed the deep inequities that still existed post-apartheid. In the park where I worked, Black and white staff performed the same jobs – yet the white workers earned double. I'll never forget the conversations I had with local women, describing how many men blamed them for infertility, how some were beaten or abandoned, and how – in tribal customs – a brother might step in to impregnate his brother's wife to save face. There was no space to acknowledge that male fertility could be a factor. In those communities, it wasn't just medical neglect, it was cultural erasure. And it struck me that this silence, in different forms, was playing out in countries everywhere – just with different languages, policies, and excuses.

That experience taught me just how critical education is. Because if we don't empower communities with accurate, respectful information – if we don't break the silence – we're not just neglecting health, we're sustaining harm.

In Japan, where the birth rate has fallen to record lows, the government has poured billions into fertility incentives and policies aimed at boosting family size – including support for IVF and childcare subsidies. Yet, male reproductive health remains an afterthought. National health campaigns largely centre on women's fertility, with public service announcements encouraging early motherhood and regular check-ups. Very few initiatives urge men to understand or improve their reproductive health. In many clinics, sperm analysis is limited to count and motility, with DNA integrity testing rarely discussed. This mirrors a global pattern where the burden of fertility is disproportionately placed on women, while male reproductive contributions remain under-analysed and under-addressed.

Denmark, one of the world's largest exporters of donor sperm, shows how even countries with advanced reproductive industries can overlook male health. While awareness of fertility science is high, education for young men about their own reproductive health is still minimal. Young men receive little education about their own fertility, despite national investment in reproductive science. The conversation rarely extends beyond donation, and testosterone decline is still considered a distant issue, not an urgent one.

In India, societal stigma around infertility disproportionately affects women, despite mounting evidence that male factor infertility accounts for half of all cases. DNA fragmentation testing is rarely offered, even in top clinics, and many couples go through repeated rounds of IVF without a full analysis of sperm quality. Education on male fertility remains minimal, and often inaccessible.

In the UAE and Saudi Arabia, clinicians are beginning to quietly raise concerns. Cultural barriers make it nearly impossible for men to speak openly about reproductive struggles. In many cases, semen sample collection is arranged with utmost discretion to preserve privacy. Despite modern medical infrastructure, deep-rooted shame continues to limit both conversation and care.

In the United States, sperm is commodified – both in the booming fertility market and in pop culture. Testosterone replacement therapy is advertised widely, and clinics promoting hormonal 'optimisation' have popped up across the country. Yet comprehensive education around male reproductive health is virtually non-existent, and many men are left unaware of the potential consequences of testosterone therapy on fertility. It's a billion-dollar industry built on quick fixes to specific symptoms, not overall health, and often without informed care.

What I've come to learn is that there are blind spots everywhere – and they're not always where you'd expect. In some countries, sperm analysis is part of routine fertility workups. In others, it's an afterthought – or not tested at all unless everything else fails. Preventative frameworks are gaining traction in pockets of Europe and Asia, where traditional medicine sometimes blends with modern lifestyle coaching. Each region seems to hold a piece of the solution, whether it's early education, culturally sensitive communication, or integrated mental health support – but these pieces rarely connect across borders. In many Western systems, the approach is still reactive: treat the problem once it's too big to ignore.

Worldwide, the average sperm count has halved in the last 50 years. Yet few countries treat this as the health crisis it is. IVF access has expanded across Europe, Asia, and the Middle East – but most programs still don't require comprehensive sperm health screening. We're trying to patch a leaking roof without ever inspecting the foundation.

Across borders, the taboos look different, but the silence feels the same. In conservative societies, the shame of discussing male fertility is cultural – a loss of masculinity. In more progressive countries, it's not shame, but apathy – a quiet assumption that men's health will take care of itself. And across both, the outcome is the same: neglect.

Right now, more organisations are rising up to support men's health – from mental wellbeing to reproductive care – but the real opportunity is connecting these efforts. A joined-up approach could turn fragmented support into a powerful preventative health movement. One focuses on mental health. Another on obesity. Another on prostate cancer. Rarely are they looking across the board at how all these systems interact – or asking why men's health is declining in so many areas at once. The dots aren't being connected, and men are the ones falling through the gaps.

Fertility sits at the intersection of all of it. It's not just a reproductive issue – it's a health issue. A public health issue. And globally, we're still not treating it as such.

I've had conversations with clinicians in Asia who are deeply concerned about declining sperm quality – but feel restricted by cultural norms that prevent them from addressing the problem openly. I've spoken to fertility specialists in the UK who say they're desperate for better male engagement tools but can't get funding to develop them. I've received DMs from men in Europe who say they're tired of being told their sperm results are 'fine' when they suspect something isn't right.

And for every frustration, there's a flicker of possibility. A progressive clinic trying something new. A school curriculum in development. A father speaking to his son differently to how his own father spoke to him. These may seem like small things. But I've learned that global change rarely starts with loud declarations. It starts with a whisper. A question. A nudge toward something better.

I remember one message from a man in Singapore. He said he and his wife had been trying for four years. After spending thousands, it was the first time someone had made him feel like his role in the process mattered. That message stayed with me.

Globally, birth rates are declining – and nations are scrambling to respond. In Australia, IVF is now being subsidised and publicly promoted, with expanded access through Medicare and state-run fertility services. Fertility medications – hormonal treatments used to support egg development during IVF – are now included on the Pharmaceutical Benefits Scheme (PBS), making treatment more affordable than ever. But nowhere in these policies is there any real push for prevention – no discussion about sperm quality, testicular health, or male hormones. It's a reactive solution that skips over half the equation.

In South Korea, the government is offering financial incentives, paternity leave, and childcare support to encourage families to grow. Singapore provides housing priority and tax rebates to larger families. In Hungary, mothers with multiple children are exempt from income tax. Israel leads the world in IVF access, offering it free to couples for their first two children. Japan, despite staggering investments in family-friendly policy, still struggles to raise its fertility rate – because policy can't override cultural hesitation, economic pressure, or silent health factors.

Innovation is also on the rise. Countries like the US and Japan are investing in technologies like in-vitro gametogenesis (IVG), artificial wombs, and lab-grown sperm – radical science that may one day redefine reproduction altogether. While cutting-edge reproduction tech is amazing, without prevention, we'll end up reliant on it, not empowered by it.

And that has consequences. These services, while life changing for many, are increasingly used as a first resort instead of a last. The more demand grows, the more it burdens already stretched healthcare systems – crowding out those who truly need it. It also reinforces the idea that medical technology can compensate for poor health habits or systemic gaps in care. It can't. Unless we start addressing the root causes – including declining sperm quality and men's overall health – the future of reproduction may be less about choice and more about reliance.

This isn't about one country or one culture. It's about building global momentum. Creating shared standards. Making space for education that's inclusive, respectful, and effective. And listening – deeply – to what men around the world are trying to tell us.

What we need is collaboration across all systems: Eastern and Western medicine, clinicians and innovators, and across generations.

Because the future of men's health won't be solved by a product alone – it will be shaped by connection, courage, and the willingness to do things differently.

We may speak different languages, follow different customs, and operate in vastly different healthcare systems. But the message is clear: men's health matters – everywhere. And it's time we started acting like it.

Your turn: share one insight from this chapter with a clinician, teacher or friend. Because real change anywhere in the world begins when we break the silence together.

Men's health matters – everywhere. And the world is finally beginning to listen.

## Putting it into practice

**For him** – Understand global gaps in care.

- Ask for more than 'normal':
    - If you're getting your sperm tested, request a full breakdown – including morphology, motility, and DNA fragmentation if possible.
    - Many men are told their results are 'normal' when they're actually far from optimal. Clarity can open conversations – and change outcomes.
    - In many countries, men with counts barely over 15 million/ml are told they're *'fine'* – yet conception often requires higher, healthier parameters (WHO, 2021).
- Challenge the silence:
    - In cultures where male reproductive health is taboo, start with safe, open questions – with a friend, a doctor, or even your partner.
    - Shifting stigma starts with small acts of courage. The more men speak, the easier it becomes for others to do the same.

- In conservative societies, clinicians have found that using neutral, accessible tools such as visual aids or patient-led education improves dialogue and reduces stigma around men's reproductive health (Alyahya et al., 2022).

**For her** – Navigate global fertility with balance.

- Don't let 'female factors' obscure the full picture:
  - Even if you've been diagnosed with PCOS or endometriosis, insist on a thorough sperm analysis as well before pursuing IVF or assisted reproduction.
  - Fertility challenges are almost never one-sided. Even with known female factors, poor sperm quality can still prevent conception or affect embryo quality.
  - Globally, half of all infertility cases involve male factors – yet many clinics still skip comprehensive sperm testing altogether (Agarwal et al., 2021).
- Learn what's normal – in your country, and beyond:
  - Educate yourself on reproductive norms and blind spots in your region – what's tested, what's ignored, and what's assumed.
  - You can't advocate for yourself if you don't know what's missing. The system won't always volunteer what you need.
  - In Japan and India, female-focused campaigns dominate public messaging about fertility – male health is often left out completely (WHO Regional Reports, 2022).

**For us** – Build global awareness, together.

- Talk to your kids about reproductive health early:
  - Wherever you live, normalise conversations about fertility, anatomy, and hormonal changes with both sons and daughters.
  - Prevention starts with education, and those values are planted long before adulthood.

- o Scandinavian countries are piloting fertility education in schools to reduce age-related infertility later in life (Gissler et al., 2020).
- Be curious about the world – and your role in it:
  - o Look beyond your own country. Follow international voices. Ask what's working elsewhere – and what we can borrow.
  - o Solutions aren't always local. Shared challenges call for shared wisdom.
  - o Countries like Israel and Hungary are leading in access to IVF – but not necessarily in prevention or education (European Society of Human Reproduction and Embryology, 2023).

## Behind the Chapter: Sources

- In many regions, especially parts of Asia and the Middle East, DNA fragmentation and full morphology testing are rarely offered unless specifically requested – leaving couples unaware of hidden sperm quality issues (Esteves et al., 2012; Agarwal et al., 2021).
- Poor sperm quality is linked to higher miscarriage rates and reduced IVF success, yet sperm testing in assisted reproduction is often basic or delayed (Zhou et al., 2021).
- Sperm health parameters can vary significantly between populations, meaning that what is considered 'normal' in one country may not be optimal in another. WHO's most recent reference values set the lower limit for sperm concentration at 15 million/ml, though conception often requires higher counts for success (WHO, 2021).
- In Japan and South Korea, large-scale public campaigns encourage early motherhood, but few target male fertility education or routine hormone testing (Shin et al., 2018; WHO Regional Reports, 2022).
- Pilot fertility education programs in Scandinavian schools show that early awareness leads to more informed health decisions and

delayed onset of age-related infertility (Hammarberg et al., 2013; Gissler et al., 2020).

- Across Europe, Australia, and the US, investment still heavily favours reactive fertility treatments over preventative approaches – a model associated with higher public health costs and delayed diagnoses (Connolly et al., 2010; Chow et al., 2021).

- Sperm counts have dropped by over 50% globally since the 1970s, with the decline now documented in Asia, Africa, and South America as well as Western countries (Levine et al., 2017; Levine et al., 2022).

- Globally, male factors account for around 50% of infertility cases – yet in many countries men are still not assessed early or comprehensively in the diagnostic process (Agarwal et al., 2021).

**CoolBeans**

# CHAPTER 23
# FOR THE CHILDREN WE'RE RAISING TODAY OR YET TO COME

**PART 1: SHAPING THE FUTURE – HEALTH, FAMILY, AND LEGACY**

I often reflect on how I can teach my children not just how to live healthy lives, but how to live with purpose, empathy, and integrity – to be responsible, loving individuals, and the kind of people who will shape a better world.

Growing up, health was a core value in my family. While we didn't always talk about it explicitly, the importance of health was evident in everything we did. One practice I hold dear from those years was the use of natural supplements, like cod liver oil, which my mother believed in wholeheartedly. My mother swore by holistic health practices, always opting for natural remedies, and only turning to medication when necessary. A spoonful of cod liver oil every morning was a cornerstone of her approach, and I see how those small acts of care have shaped my health philosophy today. These time-tested remedies, passed down through generations, remain just as relevant today. I now carry on the tradition, introducing Van and Heidi to these natural practices as part of their health journey.

Although Van and Heidi don't take cod liver oil daily, I make sure they get it during times when their immune systems need extra support. By spacing out doses, it's easier for them to tolerate, and it reduces the risk of overloading their systems, while still providing the essential nutrients they need. I've read that this approach ensures their bodies get the benefits of cod liver oil without overwhelming their systems.

This practice, rooted in a time when natural remedies were more common, continues to serve my children well today. It's a reminder that while modern medicine has its place, the value of simple, natural solutions should never be underestimated.

I was fortunate to grow up in a home where health was a consistent focus. My mother, who wasn't one for grand gestures, often said, "If your body speaks to you, listen." It's a lesson I carry with me every day. As a child, I thought it was just a saying. But as I got older, I began to truly appreciate the depth of her words. She was subtly teaching me the importance of self-care – that our bodies mirror how we treat them, and that we must listen closely, not only to the symptoms but to the deeper messages our bodies send us. I'm passing this lesson on to Van and Heidi. It's not just about telling them to eat their vegetables or take care of their bodies. It's about teaching them to listen to their own bodies, to embrace vulnerability, and to ask questions, to foster a sense of curiosity about their health and wellbeing.

I think a lot about my own experiences with health. While health was a focus in my family, reproductive health and knowledge was not. Infertility was the catalyst for this entire journey. It wasn't just about the personal struggle of conception, but about breaking a generational silence, where reproductive health, especially women's health, was kept hidden. Sharing my story was my way of opening a conversation for my children's future. For so long, we were taught to keep struggles like infertility private, to suffer in silence. But sharing my story made me realise that breaking that silence wasn't just for me, it was for the future of my children, for the families around me, and for the generations that will follow.

It's about breaking generational cycles of silence and neglect that perpetuate health struggles. As I reflect on my children, I wonder what their future will look like. Will they be able to conceive naturally when the time comes? Will they have the mental and physical strength to thrive in an ever-changing world? As parents, we hold the key to shaping that future. We have the power to equip our children with the tools they need to take control of their health – not just physically, but emotionally and mentally too.

I can't help but think of my own health journey and how it has influenced the choices I make for my family today. There was a time when I couldn't imagine the impact of one person's health on a family. But as the years have gone by, as I've learned more about male health, fertility, and the science behind our bodies, I've realised just how interconnected it all is. My own health struggles, my experiences with infertility, have shaped my passion for helping others – especially men – understand how important their health is for the future of their families.

The health of fathers plays a pivotal role in shaping their children's wellbeing, and Jordan's health decisions have had a profound impact on Van and Heidi. There's been a growing awareness around maternal health and its impact on children, but fathers have often been overlooked. I see this every day in the way Jordan takes care of himself and how his habits impact Van and Heidi. I remember a moment when Jordan decided to take his health more seriously. It was after our second miscarriage when he recognised that his mental and physical health wasn't just something that affected him – it was something that directly influenced our ability to grow our family. I admire the way he took that responsibility head-on, not just for himself but for us. Watching him now, setting an example of balance and care, is a reminder that health is something we build together. It's a legacy we pass on – not just through what we say, but through what we do.

## PART 2: PRACTICAL STEPS AND RAISING A RESILIENT GENERATION

Today we can see the growing impact of neglecting male health on children all around us. However, our family is determined not to follow this trend. I see the benefits of taking care of men's health through how Jordan's efforts are influencing the kids.

Jordan's health isn't just about him; it's about setting an example for our children to value their bodies and their mental health. Both physical and mental health are crucial for long-term wellbeing. Jordan's efforts to be mindful of his mental health, to stay active, to work through his stress and challenges – these are lessons that Van and Heidi see and absorb. They will take these lessons with them as they grow, and it will shape the way they approach their own health and wellbeing.

I value how my kids' school proactively addresses bullying. Reflecting on my own experience with bullying in primary school, I remember how I was teased in the early grades, and the solution for me was to change schools. But that shouldn't have to be the answer for every bullied child. Today, my kids are learning to manage conflict in healthier ways, to resolve issues in the playground without escalation. It's about teaching them that their emotions and experiences matter, and that the power to resolve conflict lies within them.

I'm grateful that Van and Heidi are learning to speak up for themselves and engage in constructive conversations. Lessons in emotional intelligence and resilience are just as vital as academic ones.

I want my kids to understand that they are the architects of their own future – that the choices they make today will shape who they become tomorrow. I think back to the times when Van and Heidi were learning to tie their shoes or when they first started asking me, "What's good for my body?" Those early conversations shaped how I approach teaching them about health. It's not just about telling them what foods are healthy or encouraging them to run and play. It's about teaching them to think critically, to make their own choices, and to understand that health is their responsibility.

This mission is about creating a world where health, particularly male health, is a priority. It's about making sure the world we leave treats men's health as a first though, not an afterthought. Where the next generation isn't burdened by the same health struggles we are seeing today.

My mission – my work with Cool Beans Underwear®, and my drive to improve men's health – isn't just about fertility; it's about legacy. It's about creating a healthier future for everyone, starting with my children and extending to every man, woman, and child on this planet. It's about breaking the cycles of poor health, poor communication, and poor education. It's about building a future where health is a priority, not a secondary concern.

The ripple effect is real. One conversation, one act of courage, can transform how we view health and legacy. It wasn't easy for me to open up, but when I did, I began to see the ripple effects in the conversations I had with friends, with family, and with strangers. People started sharing their own experiences – men, women, parents, and even those without children – about how their health had been misunderstood or neglected. It became clear: this isn't just my fight, it's our fight – a fight for all families, children, and generations. And with each conversation, we're building a world where health isn't an afterthought, but a priority.

Our world is changing rapidly. From the food we eat to the technology we use, our way of life is evolving, fundamentally altering our biology and health. These changes aren't just impacting us today; they're shaping our children's future. As parents, we must understand how these changes are affecting their health and what we can do to protect them.

Our diets are increasingly filled with processed foods, much of which is packaged in plastics containing Bisphenol A (BPA), a substance linked to hormonal disruption. While manufacturers have moved away from BPA, the question remains: what are they replacing it with? Alternatives like Bisphenol S (BPS) and Bisphenol F (BPF) still pose potential risks, potentially disrupting our endocrine system. Along with plastics, microplastics – tiny plastic particles found in oceans, air, and food – are now present in most of our food items, from seafood to table salt. These particles, though invisible, are absorbed by our bodies, and their long-term effects on human health remain unclear.

As a family, we can take small but significant steps to reduce our exposure to microplastics. First, try to avoid bottled water and use a reusable water bottle instead. The plastic used in bottles can degrade over time, releasing microplastics into the water. Next, reduce your consumption of seafood, as marine life is one of the biggest culprits in microplastic contamination. Finally, consider using a water filter to help reduce the amount of microplastics in your tap water. While we can't completely eliminate microplastics from our lives, we can take actions to reduce our exposure.

In today's world, technology is a constant presence. Wi-Fi signals, Bluetooth devices, and electromagnetic fields (EMFs) are now part of everyday life. While we can't avoid technology, we do need to be mindful of how these technologies may be impacting our health. There is ongoing research into how EMFs, which are emitted by devices like smartphones, Wi-Fi routers, and Bluetooth-enabled products, might affect our biological systems.

Unfortunately, technology is a part of our daily lives, and I know that like most kids today, Van and Heidi are on screens too much. That's why I place such a high value on the times when we can disconnect and go camping or hiking. For us, these moments in nature, away from technology, are essential. The ability to be one with nature, to breathe in fresh air, and to engage with the environment around us without distraction is vital for their development – and for all of us as a family.

We can't deny that technology is a huge part of our future, and it's going to be critical for their success in the workforce, especially as AI and new technologies become central to the world they'll enter. But it's just as important to give them the opportunity to unplug and reconnect with the world around them. We've come to realise that technology is rewiring our brains, especially for kids, making it harder for them to focus for long periods. Being able to disconnect and fully immerse ourselves in nature allows their brains to reset, to refocus, and to truly be present. These breaks from technology are crucial for their mental health and wellbeing.

Some studies suggest that long-term exposure to EMFs could have a detrimental impact on sperm quality, as well as other aspects of health such as hormone regulation and brain function. The growing reliance on technology means that many of us are constantly surrounded by these electromagnetic fields, which may be contributing to the overall decline in male fertility.

As parents, we need to be mindful of how technology is impacting our children's health. Limiting screen time, especially before bedtime, is one way to reduce exposure to EMFs. Encouraging outdoor play, physical activity, and a balanced lifestyle can help mitigate some of the negative effects of technology on our health. And, of course, talking to our kids about healthy technology habits is an important part of future-proofing their wellbeing.

As we look to the future, it's clear that the choices we make today will have lasting effects on our children's health. The way we eat, the technology we use, and the environment we live in all contribute to their biology and wellbeing. And the reality is, the world they will inherit will be vastly different from the one we grew up in.

While I have juggled the demands of writing this book, scaling Cool Beans Underwear®, and a busy family life, Jordan has really stepped up as the primary parent in many ways. One of the things he's taken over is cooking healthy, hearty meals for dinner. It's been so important for us as parents to show our kids the value of home cooking, and it's something we've worked hard to instill in them. But it's not just about cooking for them; it's about involving them in the process.

We make it a point to let Van and Heidi help pick out new ingredients at the grocery store. While it's important not to consume too much seafood, the seafood counter at Woolworths is a particular highlight for the kids. The kids can get excited about trying things like fish heads, lobster tails, or new recipes with prawns. It's a fun, hands-on way to introduce them to healthy foods while also teaching them the value of knowing where their food comes from and how to prepare it.

Taking them to fresh food markets, where they can see the raw ingredients and get excited about cooking with them, has been an amazing way to broaden their culinary interests. It gives them ownership over the food they eat and fosters an interest in nutrition that I hope will stay with them for the rest of their lives.

I often reflect on one of my favourite holidays as a child, a memory that still stands out after all these years. When I was around 10, my parents took me skiing in the Australian Snowy Mountains. They made sure we experienced the area in a variety of ways, staying in different accommodations each time. But the most memorable trip was when we stayed at the bottom of the range in a fully off-grid house. It had no electricity, no hot water – we had to light a fire to cook and heat the water. And yet it remains one of the best experiences I've ever had.

The house was small, cozy, and warm, but what stood out most was the silence. There were no screens, no distractions; just us, the fire, the mountains, and the sound of a stream running in the background. We spent the evenings playing cards, reading stories, and simply being present with each other. In a world full of technology and constant connection, it's hard to imagine the kind of peace we had there. But it's this kind of experience that I want to give my children – a chance to disconnect and be fully present, to appreciate the simple things, and to create memories that will last a lifetime.

One thing we do know is that health systems will need to evolve. We can no longer rely on the same outdated models of healthcare that treat symptoms after the fact. Instead, we need preventative healthcare models that focus on understanding and mitigating the risks of our changing world. This includes addressing issues like poor diet, sedentary lifestyles, environmental toxins, and the overuse of technology.

As parents, we can take proactive steps today to ensure that our children have the tools, knowledge, and support to navigate these challenges. It starts with education, instilling healthy habits, and fostering open conversations about the importance of both physical and mental health. But it also means advocating for change, both within our families and in the broader health systems.

When I look at my children, I feel a deep responsibility to not just care for them in the present, but to ensure they have the tools to navigate the future. We may not have all the answers yet, but one thing I know for sure: if we don't start making these changes now, the health of future generations will be at risk.

One of the best ways we've been able to give Van and Heidi a healthy experience is through our yearly camping trips to Moreton Island. We get on the ferry, leave everything behind, and set up camp in complete isolation. It's one of their favourite holidays, and I can see why. For 10 days, there's no technology, no screens, just the simplicity of nature. The kids call it their 'happy place', and I can't help but agree with them.

There's something powerful about stepping away from the chaos of daily life and returning to the basics. Cooking over an open fire, going on long walks, and playing games together without any distractions –

it's during these moments that we can truly connect, and that's when I see how much my kids grow, both emotionally and physically. These trips remind us of the importance of being fully present with each other, something I'm committed to giving them as they grow.

Ultimately, the future of health isn't just about surviving – it's about thriving. It's about creating a world where our children can live long, healthy lives, free from the limitations we face today. We may not have all the answers yet, but I know one thing: it starts with us.

The future of health is in our hands. And with every small change we make today, we are building a foundation for a healthier tomorrow. When I look at my children, I see more than just my legacy. I see the changes they're already making, the way they learn to care for themselves, and the way they challenge the norms around them. I see hope for a future that's different from the one we grew up in – a future where health is truly at the centre of everything. Every small decision we make today, every conversation we have about health, every action we take to break old cycles, is building a world where health, wellbeing, and love are the foundation for everything. That's the world I hope to leave behind. And that's the world I believe we will create – together.

This journey is not just mine, it's all of ours. Together, we can create a healthier, more resilient future for our children, where health is not an afterthought but the foundation for everything they do.

## Putting it into practice

**For him** – Empower our sons to thrive.

- Cultivate emotional intelligence:
    - Start open conversations with your son about emotions, stress, and vulnerability, teaching him that vulnerability is a strength, not a weakness.

- - This teaches your son the importance of emotional resilience, which is essential for mental and emotional health throughout life.
  - Studies show that emotional intelligence in boys is linked to better mental health outcomes and stronger relationships (Goleman, 1995).
- Teach resilience through action:
  - Empower your son to face challenges with a growth mindset. Teach him how to problem-solve and make decisions through trial and error.
  - Building resilience equips your son with the ability to cope with life's ups and downs, fostering long-term mental strength.
  - Research indicates that children with resilience are more likely to become emotionally stable adults (Masten, 2001).

**For her** – Raise daughters who understand health.

- Support her emotional growth:
  - Teach your daughter how to manage her emotions through mindfulness, journaling, or talking openly about her feelings.
  - Emotional intelligence enables your daughter to manage stress and anxiety, enhancing her ability to navigate challenges with balance.
  - Emotional wellbeing is linked to better academic performance and mental health outcomes in young women (Eisenberg & Lennon, 1983).
- Encourage strong, independent health choices:
  - Teach your daughter about her body, her reproductive health, and how to make informed health decisions from a young age.
  - Empowering her with knowledge about her body builds confidence and autonomy, setting her up for healthier future choices.

- Research shows that early education on reproductive health leads to better health outcomes and fewer reproductive issues later in life (Tiggemann & Slater, 2014).

**For us** – Strengthen family health together.

- Create family rituals around healthy living:
  - Involve the whole family in meal planning and preparation, making healthy eating fun and inclusive. Make outdoor activities a regular part of the family routine.
  - Family participation in cooking and exercise fosters healthier habits, boosts physical health, and strengthens family bonds.
  - Studies show that family-based interventions around physical activity and healthy eating improve children's health outcomes, including weight control (Golan & Crow, 2004).
- Model healthy boundaries:
  - Practice and model how to set healthy boundaries with time, technology, and social interactions. Encourage your children to set their own boundaries for self-care.
  - Setting boundaries promotes mental health and reduces stress, empowering your children to prioritise their own wellbeing.
  - Setting boundaries has been shown to increase emotional satisfaction and life satisfaction (Harris & Harris, 2018).

**For us all** – Create a legacy of wellness.

- Practice gratitude as a family:
  - Make it a daily family ritual to share three things you're grateful for, fostering a positive mindset in your home.
  - Practicing gratitude strengthens family bonds, improves mental health, and builds resilience.
  - Research shows that gratitude practices significantly increase happiness and emotional wellbeing (Emmons & McCullough, 2003).

- Embrace nature's healing power:
  - Commit to regular outdoor family activities, such as hiking, walking, or simply spending time in nature.
  - Nature exposure helps reduce stress, improve mood, and strengthen immunity for the whole family.
  - Studies indicate that spending time in nature lowers cortisol levels and improves focus and overall wellbeing (Barton et al., 2009).

## Behind the chapter: Sources

- Studies show that exposure to BPA, often found in food packaging, can disrupt endocrine function, leading to negative impacts on fertility and hormone regulation (Vandenberg et al., 2012).
- Microplastics have been detected in human tissue, and studies suggest they may contribute to inflammation, gut dysfunction, and hormone disruption over time (Prata et al., 2020).
- Research has found that prolonged exposure to electromagnetic fields (EMFs) from mobile devices and Wi-Fi can affect sperm motility, morphology, and DNA fragmentation (Agarwal et al., 2011).
- Male mental and physical health have been found to directly impact children's wellbeing, with studies indicating that poor paternal health correlates with an increased risk of behavioural and emotional issues in children (Miller et al., 2009).
- Early reproductive health education has been shown to improve young people's health literacy, leading to better long-term health decisions and reduced infertility rates (Hammarberg et al., 2013).
- The decisions made by parents, particularly related to diet and lifestyle, have a lasting impact on the health of their children, with intergenerational effects on both fertility and general wellbeing (Barker et al., 2008).

- A growing body of research supports the notion that fathers' health choices, including mental and physical wellbeing, significantly influence their children's development and overall health (Fleming et al., 2018).
- Encouraging resilience and emotional intelligence in children has been shown to lead to better long-term mental health outcomes and stronger relationships in adulthood (Goleman, 1995; Masten, 2001).
- Teaching children about healthy boundaries has been linked to improved emotional satisfaction, life satisfaction, and stress management (Harris & Harris, 2018).
- Nature exposure has been shown to lower cortisol levels, improve focus, and strengthen immunity for both children and adults (Barton et al., 2009).
- Family-based interventions that focus on healthy eating and physical activity have been shown to improve children's health outcomes, including weight control and long-term wellbeing (Golan & Crow, 2004).

## THIS SIDE OF THE STORY
## – A WORLD WE ARE CREATING FOR OUR CHILDREN
## – AND ALL OF US

As I sit here, reflecting on everything shared in these pages, I realise something deeply important. This mission isn't just about me or even just about my children. It's about all of us – the world we're building today for future generations.

If you're a parent, you've already been part of the conversation. Your choices shape the lives of your children. But what if you're not a parent yet? Or maybe you've already raised your kids? You're still incredibly important in this mission. Whether you have nephews, nieces, godchildren, or mentor children – your role in shaping the future of the next generation matters deeply.

We all have influence over the young people in our lives, and we all play a part in how they grow, learn, and understand their health. The truth is the mission of building a healthier future is not one that can be carried by just a few – it requires all of us.

If you're someone who doesn't yet have children, you can still drive this change by offering guidance to those who do. By being a role model. By supporting the parents around you, whether they're family or friends, in the choices they make for their children. You can be a part of this movement by showing up in big and small ways for the next generation.

Every decision we make to support better health, every conversation we have with the young people around us about their mental, emotional, and physical health – we are contributing to a ripple effect. The health of one person influences a whole network – from parents to extended families, friends to colleagues. It's a movement that touches many lives, and no one person can do it alone.

So, whether you're raising your own children or mentoring others, know that your actions matter. You are part of something much bigger. The changes we need, the shifts in health we need to see, won't come from one person – they start with all of us. Together, we can raise a generation that values health and wellbeing, understands the importance of living with purpose, and connects with others in meaningful ways.

As we create this healthier world for our children, we're creating it for all of us – for the future we share. It's up to each of us to step up and drive this change. Because in the end, we're all shaping the world our children will inherit.

> Dear children,
>
> I'm writing this letter to you because I believe in the future you'll create. I believe you have the power to shape the world in ways we can't even imagine yet. The choices you make today will lay the foundation for that future.
>
> Your health isn't just about eating vegetables or going to the doctor when you're sick. It's about listening to your body, understanding how you feel, and taking care of yourself – not just for today, but for tomorrow. Your health is the most important thing you can care for because it's what will carry you through life.
>
> But there's something even bigger than that. It's about the world you'll help create. The earth, the animals, the plants, the people – all of it is connected. Just like you care for your own health, you'll need to care for the health of the world around you. It's not just about looking after yourself; it's about understanding that the choices we make for the planet, for others, and for ourselves all matter.

## For the children we're raising today or yet to come

There's a world waiting for you to make it better. A world where we live together, in harmony, with nature and with each other. Where health isn't something we talk about when things go wrong, but something we celebrate and nurture every single day. And you – yes, you – will help make that world a reality.

So, take care of yourself. Listen to your body, treat it with love and respect, and remember that it's okay to ask for help when you need it. And when you grow up and become parents, mentors, and leaders – I hope you'll pass on these lessons. Teach the next generation to care for their health, respect nature, and look after each other.

The world you inherit and the world you leave behind – they're both in your hands. I believe in you, and I believe you'll make it better than we ever could.

With hope and love,
Saara X

**CoolBeans**

## EPILOGUE
# THE MISSION IS JUST BEGINNING

Closing this book, I am filled with gratitude for how far we've come, and with an unwavering fire for the journey still ahead. What began with my personal struggles has blossomed into something far bigger – a movement that transcends my story to encompass families, communities, and ultimately, the health of our future generations.

What started with the goal of improving men's health – addressing the silent suffering, the under-discussed pain, and the neglected aspects of male wellbeing – has grown into a broader mission: to future-proof natural conception, to reduce sperm health decline, and to create healthier families for a healthier tomorrow. The road ahead is long, but the momentum is building, and the work we are doing today will have ripple effects for generations to come.

We are expanding our mission, extending beyond Cool Beans Underwear® into education, policy, and community outreach. It's about shifting the conversation around men's health and starting a global dialogue that embraces not just physical health, but mental health, reproductive health, and ultimately, the health of our children. We can't make real transformation without education, awareness, and advocacy – these are the cornerstones of what we're building.

We're starting with awareness, as without awareness, change cannot occur. As we grow, so too will our reach and our ability to create real, lasting change. The future of men's health isn't just about solving the issues we see today. It's about creating a culture that is proactive, that values men's health as a foundational element of family health, and that works to eliminate the stigma and silence that surrounds it.

We'll evolve by forging alliances with medical societies, campaigning for male health policies, and launching grassroots fertility-awareness events in every region, to help normalise the conversation about male fertility, sperm health, and mental wellbeing.

But this journey isn't just about raising awareness for today; it's about transforming the world we're building for tomorrow, creating policy change and bringing government and those with power to make change into the conversation. The rise of technology and innovation, while providing us with many conveniences, also creates new health challenges. We're becoming more sedentary, consuming more processed foods, and facing environmental toxins – all of which directly impact our wellbeing. As we continue to progress in this digital age, we must evolve our approach to health and wellness. This isn't a five- or ten-year mission. This is an ongoing journey, one that requires us all to make small, intentional changes every day.

Together, we can create a future in which our children grow up in a world where health – physical, mental, and reproductive health – is prioritised. A future where natural conception is not something we fight to preserve, but something that is taken for granted because we've laid the groundwork today to ensure our kids have the healthiest start to life possible. By addressing the decline in men's health now, we're setting the foundation for a healthier tomorrow – a tomorrow where our children inherit a world that values health as its cornerstone.

## Epilogue: The mission is just beginning

If you've made it this far, I want to take a moment to thank you. Thank you for reading, for committing to understanding the challenges men face, and for joining me on this journey. Your dedication to improving men's health and future-proofing natural conception is not just admirable – it's essential. Your willingness to be part of this movement, to help shift the conversation, and to make a difference is what will truly transform the future.

This is your movement too.

I'm inviting you to join me on this mission. Become part of the movement working to shift the narrative, change the conversation, and make men's health a priority for all of us. Together, we can create a world where fertility isn't a struggle, where health is a right, not a privilege, and where our future is one of wellbeing, strength, and resilience.

Share the story. Support the mission. Be a part of the movement. Because the work we start today will shape the world they inherit tomorrow.

Find out more and to follow the impact we're creating, join our community at: coolbeansunderwear.com

**CoolBeans**

**READER REFLECTION**

# WHAT WILL YOU LEAVE BEHIND?

*If nothing changes today, what will the world look like in 10 years? In 20? Now, think about the impact your actions can have on shifting that future. How can you be part of that change?*

**YOUR TURN**

As you reach the end of this book, it's time to reflect on your own role in this mission. This is not just about me – it's about all of us, no matter who we are or where we come from. Now, it's time for you to think about the legacy you want to leave and how you can be a part of the movement to change the conversation about health and the future.

## WHAT LEGACY DO YOU WANT TO LEAVE BEHIND FOR THE NEXT GENERATION?

*"I want my children, and all children, to grow up in a world where they understand the importance of health from a young age, and know they have the power to shape their futures. My legacy is to raise a generation that is not afraid to talk about their health, whether mental, physical, or reproductive." – Saara*

**Write it down:**

## WHAT CONVERSATIONS ARE YOU NOW READY TO START?

*"I'm ready to start talking openly about men's health, breaking the silence around infertility, mental health, and the importance of self-care. It's time we make these conversations part of the norm, especially for our children, boys and girls alike." – Saara*

**Write it down:**

## WHAT ACTION CAN YOU TAKE TODAY TO CONTRIBUTE TO THIS MISSION?

*"I will continue to educate myself and my community about the importance of men's health and start normalising these conversations with my friends, family, and social media. I will also make sure my children understand the importance of their own health and encourage them to make it a priority from a young age." – Saara*

**Write it down:**

## Reader Reflection: What will you leave behind?

**HOW CAN YOU MAKE HEALTH A PRIORITY IN YOUR OWN LIFE AND COMMUNITY?**

*"By taking care of my own health, both mental and physical, I set an example for others. I will continue advocating for healthier lifestyles in my family, my work, and my community, making sure that men and women, boys and girls, feel empowered to look after themselves." – Saara*

**Write it down:**

## WHAT CHANGES WILL YOU MAKE TO FUTURE-PROOF THE HEALTH OF THE NEXT GENERATION?

*"I will teach my children to value their health and ask questions about their bodies, to avoid harmful health patterns, and to start young in protecting their fertility and wellbeing. I also hope to encourage everyone to consider the impact of our choices – from diet to lifestyle to mental health – on the future."* – Saara

**Write it down:**

## Reader Reflection: What will you leave behind?

## TAKE ACTION

- **Share it with someone**: Talking about your reflections can solidify your commitment to this mission and help inspire others.

- **Let it change how you show up tomorrow**: Let your reflections guide how you approach your health, your conversations, and your actions going forward.

The power to create change starts with us. Together, we can transform the future.

## INCLUSIVITY NOTE:

Whether or not you have children, whether you are a man or a woman, young or old – this movement is for you. Men's health affects everyone. The ripple effect of healthy choices and conversations will impact future generations – including daughters, sons, friends, and partners – no matter who you are. Join the movement. Make a difference. Together, we'll create a healthier tomorrow.

**CoolBeans**

**BONUS SECTION**

# TOOLS FOR CHANGE-MAKERS

For readers, partners, educators, and clinicians who want to take the next step.

## 1. TOP FIVE ACTIONS TO SUPPORT MEN'S HEALTH TODAY

Making small, intentional changes can have a significant impact on both men's health and the future of natural conception. Here's how you can take action today:

- **Wear Cool Beans Underwear® every day.**
  To reduce scrotal heat, prioritise breathable, anatomical underwear that supports your fertility, hormone regulation, and overall health. Cool Beans Underwear® is specifically designed to reduce heat, promote circulation, and protect testicular health. With Cool Beans, you're investing in your long-term wellbeing – it's the only purpose-designed underwear to reduce heat and support testicular health.
  **Start today – make the change and wear Cool Beans Underwear®.**

- **Start the conversation.**
  Talk to the men in your life – brothers, partners, sons, dads. Ask them how they're really feeling. Opening up about mental and physical health starts the process of breaking down the barriers around men's health.

- **Normalise check-ups.**
  Sperm testing, hormone panels, testicular checks – prevention starts with awareness. Encourage the men in your life to prioritise their health by getting regular check-ups.

- **Lead by example.**
  Every small change you make toward better health makes it easier for someone else to speak up and follow suit. Be the change you want to see in the world.

- **Support your health in everyday actions.**
  Avoid prolonged sitting, hot car seats, and warm laps with laptops or pets. These seemingly small changes, when combined with wearing Cool Beans, can make a big difference in long-term health.

## 2. PRACTITIONER AND CLINICIAN QUICK GUIDE
### Why clinicians are recommending Cool Beans Underwear®:

- **Post-operative scrotal support**
  Useful for hernia, vasectomy, testicular/prostate surgery, penile, scrotal, and urological surgeries.

- **Management of hot flushes after chemotherapy or hormone treatment.**
  Cool Beans Underwear® helps manage hot flushes by using the natural cooling properties of the scrotal vascular system. The design promotes blood flow and temperature regulation, helping the body rid itself of excess heat, particularly beneficial for patients undergoing chemotherapy or hormone treatments who experience hot flushes.

- **Testosterone optimisation**
Testosterone levels are declining globally, affecting men's physical, mental, and reproductive health. By improving testosterone levels, we help optimise the balance of all other hormones, which is essential for maintaining energy, retaining muscle mass, cognitive alertness, and overall wellbeing. Cool Beans Underwear® helps maintain optimal scrotal temperature, which is essential for preserving testosterone production and supporting long-term hormonal health.

- **Preventative support in fertility and ART (Assisted Reproductive Technologies)**
Whether trying for natural conception or undergoing IVF, Cool Beans Underwear® helps improve sperm health by regulating scrotal temperature, which is crucial for healthy sperm production. By supporting sperm health, Cool Beans improves conception rates, reduces miscarriage incidence, and ultimately contributes to healthier children. The design supports men's fertility journeys, whether in natural conception or ART procedures, by optimising sperm quality and overall reproductive health.

- **Groin skin conditions**
Helps reduce irritation and conditions caused by friction or heat in the groin area. Cool Beans Underwear® promotes comfort and reduces the risk of chafing, rashes, and other skin conditions in sensitive areas.

- **Pelvic floor support**
Provides added support for the pelvic region, beneficial for general health and post-surgical recovery. The anatomical design provides extra stability for those recovering from pelvic or groin injuries.

- **Support for torn muscles within the groin area**
Offers gentle support for recovery from muscle strains or injuries in the groin. Cool Beans Underwear® helps stabilise the area and provides relief, aiding in the healing process.

- **Varicocele management**
Assists in reducing discomfort and supporting the affected veins in the scrotal area. Cool Beans Underwear® helps to improve circulation and reduce pressure on the veins, making it beneficial for managing varicocele symptoms.

- **Mental health**
Testosterone plays a crucial role in mental health. The lower your testosterone levels, the more susceptible you are to mental health issues such as depression, anxiety, and stress. The better your testosterone levels are, the easier it becomes to manage these issues, should they arise. Cool Beans Underwear® helps maintain optimal testosterone levels, which supports mental resilience, stress reduction, and overall emotional wellbeing.

- **Longevity**
Supports long-term scrotal health, which is critical for maintaining healthy testosterone levels. The better the testosterone levels, the better men will age, with improved muscle mass retention, cognitive alertness, and overall vitality as they age. Cool Beans Underwear® helps create a foundation for healthier aging by promoting optimal hormone balance.

- **Sexual performance and desire**
The better your testosterone, the better your sexual performance and desire. Cool Beans Underwear® helps maintain optimal temperature and support, improving sexual health by reducing testicular heat. Additionally, by offering proper scrotal support, it improves blood flow to all parts of the genitalia, enhancing sexual performance. Results are typically seen around 2 months after consistent use of Cool Beans.

- **Athlete mental and physical performance**
While Cool Beans Underwear® is not intended for high-intensity sports, it is ideal for activities like gym workouts, hiking, or walking. By reducing the compounding effects of testicular heat when at

rest, Cool Beans optimises testosterone levels, which are essential for both physical and mental performance. During a sports season, prolonged exposure to testicular heat can significantly reduce testosterone levels, as the testes don't fully recover between physical exertion. This decline can lead to diminished athletic performance, both physically and mentally, as the season progresses. Cool Beans helps athletes manage their recovery during the off-season and reduce the long-term effects of heat exposure during the playing season.

- **Testicular pain**
  Provides relief from general testicular pain, often caused by inadequate scrotal support, heat, inflammation, or strain. Cool Beans Underwear® offers optimal support, reducing discomfort associated with poor support or excessive heat. This helps alleviate testicular pain by ensuring the testes are positioned correctly, allowing for better circulation and reducing strain. Whether from daily activities or sports, Cool Beans helps provide the comfort and support needed for recovery and long-term health.

**Sample request link:** coolbeansunderwear.com/clinicians

## 3. RESOURCES AND FURTHER READING

Want to learn more?
Want to share your story?
Visit: coolbeansunderwear.com

Want Saara to speak at your event, school, or organisation?
Contact: hello@coolbeansunderwear.com

## 4. JOIN THE MOVEMENT

It's time to take action, be part of the conversation, and contribute to the mission that's changing the future of men's health. Here's how you can get involved:

- Follow @coolbeansunderwear on Instagram, Facebook, and LinkedIn
- Use the hashtag #CoolChangeMovement

**Get involved:**

- Support campaigns for earlier hormone and sperm screening in young men.
- Share your story to shift stigma and silence.
- Connect your clinic, workplace, or school to our educational programs.
- Become a partner or donor to expand this critical work.

## THANK YOU FOR JOINING THE MISSION

You've already taken a significant step by reading this book and engaging with the ideas within it. But now, the work continues – and we need you. By joining the movement, sharing the story, and supporting the mission, you're helping to create a future where men's health is a priority, not an afterthought. This is not just about individual health – this is about the health of families, communities, and future generations. Together, we can change the conversation, create a lasting impact, and ultimately build a healthier tomorrow.

# REFERENCES

- AAP Council on Sports Medicine & Fitness. (2019). Sports safety and protective equipment guidance.
- Abbasi, B., Kimiagar, M., Sadeghniiat, K., Shirazi, M. M., Hedayati, M., & Rashidkhani, B. (2012). The effect of magnesium supplementation on primary insomnia in elderly: A double-blind placebo-controlled clinical trial. *Journal of Research in Medical Sciences, 17*(12), 1161-1169.
- Addis, M. E., & Mahalik, J. R. (2003). Men, masculinity, and the contexts of help seeking. *American Psychologist, 58*(1), 5-14.
- Agarwal, A., Baskaran, S., Parekh, N., et al. (2021). Male infertility. *The Lancet, 397*(10271), 319-333.
- Agarwal, A., Desai, N. R., Makker, K., Varghese, A., Mouradi, R., Sabanegh, E., & Sharma, R. (2008). Effects of radiofrequency electromagnetic waves (RF-EMW) from cell phones on human ejaculated semen: An in vitro pilot study. *Fertility and Sterility, 89*(1), 124-128.
- Agarwal, A., Desai, N. R., Makker, K., Varghese, A., Mouradi, R., Sabanegh, E., & Sharma, R. (2015). Male factor infertility: A clinical guide to the evaluation and management. *European Urology, 67*(6), 1160-1175. https://doi.org/10.1016/j.eururo.2015.01.001
- Agarwal, A., Gupta, S., & Sharma, R. (2014). Oxidative stress and its implications in female infertility. *Reproductive BioMedicine Online.*

- Agarwal, A., Gupta, S., & Sharma, R. K. (2014). Role of oxidative stress in female reproduction. *Reproductive Biology and Endocrinology, 3*(28). https://doi.org/10.1186/1477-7827-3-28
- Agarwal, A., Mulgund, A., & Hamada, A. (2015). A unique view on male infertility: A comprehensive review. *Fertility and Sterility, 103*(6), 1194-1215.
- Agarwal, A., Mulgund, A., Hamada, A., & Chyatte, M. R. (2015). A unique view on male infertility around the globe. *Reproductive Biology and Endocrinology, 13*(1), 37. https://doi.org/10.1186/s12958-015-0032-1
- Agarwal, A., Mulgund, A., Hamada, A., & Chyatte, M. R. (2015). A unique view on male infertility around the globe. *Reproductive Biology and Endocrinology, 13*(1), 37. https://doi.org/10.1186/s12958-015-0032-1
- Agarwal, A., Mullen, J. B., & Al-Dakheel, M. A. (2011). Effect of mobile phone usage on sperm motility and morphology: A systematic review and meta-analysis. *Asian Journal of Andrology, 13*(1), 31-39.
- AIHW. (2022). *Australia's Children: Mental health*. Australian Institute of Health and Welfare.
- Aitken, R. J., & Baker, H. W. G. (2006). Sperm DNA fragmentation and its relationship to infertility. *Human Reproduction Update, 12*(3), 213-224.
- Aitken, R. J., Gibb, Z., & Lambourne, S. R. (2019). The effects of oxidative stress on male fertility. *Reproductive Biomedicine Online, 39*(6), 684-695. https://doi.org/10.1016/j.rbmo.2019.08.004
- Allen, S. M., & Hawkins, A. J. (1999). Maternal gatekeeping: Mothers' beliefs and behaviors that inhibit greater father involvement. *Journal of Marriage and Family, 61*(1), 199-212.
- American Society for Reproductive Medicine (ASRM). (2015). *Guidance on fertility preservation in women of reproductive age*.
- American Society of Clinical Oncology. (2018). Fertility preservation for patients with cancer: ASCO clinical practice guideline update. *Journal of Clinical Oncology, 36*(19), 1994-2001. https://doi.org/10.1200/JCO.2018.78.1914

# References

- Andersen, M. L., Tufik, S., & Mello, M. T. (2016). Sleep and male reproductive health: A review of the literature. *International Journal of Endocrinology, 2016*, 1-8.
- Anderson, K., Nisenblat, V., & Norman, R. (2010). Lifestyle factors in people seeking infertility treatment - A review. *Australian and New Zealand Journal of Obstetrics and Gynaecology*.
- ASRM (American Society for Reproductive Medicine). (2015). *Fertility and age: The impact of age on fertility in both men and women*. Retrieved from www.asrm.org
- Baazeem, A., Al-Shaiji, T., & Shammari, S. (2011). Male infertility: Male reproductive health. *Andrology, 1*(4), 227-234.
- Baazeem, A., et al. (2011). Male infertility and the role of sperm quality in assisted reproductive technology. *Asian Journal of Andrology, 13*(5), 619-628.
- Baetens, P., et al. (2016). Psychosocial impact of donor conception: A narrative review. *Human Reproduction Update, 22*(6), 737-747.
- Bandura, A. (1977). *Social Learning Theory*. Englewood Cliffs, NJ: Prentice Hall.
- Barker, D. J. P., & Osmond, C. (2008). Fetal origins of coronary heart disease. *British Medical Journal, 307*(6902), 245-248.
- Barton, J., Hine, R., & Pretty, J. (2009). The health benefits of walking in greenspace: A systematic review of the evidence. *International Journal of Environmental Health Research, 19*(3), 248-267.
- Basaria, S. (2014). Male hypogonadism. *The Lancet, 383*(9924), 1250-1263.
- Baumrind, D. (1991). The influence of parenting style on adolescent competence and substance use. *Journal of Early Adolescence, 11*(1), 56-95. https://doi.org/10.1177/0272431691111004
- Bentov, Y., Yavorska, T., Esfandiari, N., et al. (2014). The use of mitochondrial nutrients to improve oocyte and embryo quality: A review of the literature and future directions. *Journal of Assisted Reproduction and Genetics, 31*(6), 689-695.

- Blomberg Jensen, M. (2014). Vitamin D and male reproduction. *Nature Reviews Endocrinology*.
- Bögels, S. M., Lehtonen, A., & Restifo, K. (2014). Mindful parenting in mental health care. *Mindfulness, 5*, 536-551.
- Cancer Research UK. (2022). Testicular cancer-signs and symptoms; getting to know what's normal.
- Chaplin, T. M., & Aldao, A. (2013). Gender differences in emotion expression in children: A meta-analytic review. *Psychological Bulletin, 139*(4), 735-765.
- Chavarro, J. E., Rich-Edwards, J. W., Rosner, B. A., & Willett, W. C. (2006). Iron intake and risk of ovulatory infertility. *Obstetrics & Gynecology, 108*(5), 1145-1152.
- Chavarro, J. E., Rich-Edwards, J. W., Rosner, B. A., & Willett, W. C. (2007). Diet and lifestyle in the prevention of ovulatory disorder infertility. *Obstetrics & Gynecology, 110*(5), 1050-1058. https://doi.org/10.1097/01.AOG.0000287293.25465.e1
- Chavarro, J.E., Rich-Edwards, J.W., Rosner, B.A., & Willett, W.C., (2007). Dietary fatty acid intakes and the risk of ovulatory infertility. *American Journal of Clinical Nutrition, 85*(1), 231-237. https://doi.org/10.1093/ajcn/85.1.231
- Chiu, Y. H., Afeiche, M. C., Gaskins, A. J., Williams, P. L., Mendiola, J., Jørgensen, N., ... & Chavarro, J. E. (2014). Sugar-sweetened beverage intake in relation to semen quality and reproductive hormone levels in young men. *Human Reproduction, 29*(7), 1575-1584. https://doi.org/10.1093/humrep/deu102
- Chow, E. J., Cakmak, H., Rosen, M. P., & Cedars, M. I. (2021). Cost-effectiveness of reproductive health interventions: A systematic review. *Fertility and Sterility, 115*(1), 12-25.
- Colagar, A. H., Marzony, E. T., & Chaichi, M. J. (2009). Zinc levels in seminal plasma are associated with sperm quality in fertile and infertile men. *Nutrition Research*.
- Conde-Agudelo, A., & Díaz-Rossello, J. L. (2016). Kangaroo mother care to reduce morbidity and mortality in low birthweight infants. *Cochrane Database of Systematic Reviews, 2016*(8), CD002771. https://doi.org/10.1002/14651858.CD002771.pub4

# References

- Connolly, M. P., Hoorens, S., & Chambers, G. M. (2010). The costs and consequences of assisted reproductive technology: An economic perspective. *Human Reproduction Update, 16*(6), 603-613.
- Costabile, R. A. (2007). Chronic testicular pain: Evaluation and management. *Urologic Clinics of North America, 34*(2), 267-276.
- Costabile, R. A. (2007). Idiopathic testicular pain: Pathophysiology and treatment. *Urology, 70*(6), 1104-1108.
- Courtenay, W. H. (2000). Constructions of masculinity and their influence on men's well-being: A theory of gender and health. *Social Science & Medicine, 50*(10), 1385-1401.
- Crinnion, W. J. (2010). Components of practical clinical detox programs-sauna as a therapeutic tool. *Alternative Medicine Review, 15*(3), 215-225.
- Dasgupta, N., & Asgari, S. (2004). Seeing is believing: Exposure to counterstereotypic women leaders... *Journal of Experimental Social Psychology, 40*(5), 642-658.
- Domar, A. D., & Lasky, R. (1993). The psychological impact of infertility treatment. *Fertility and Sterility, 59*(4), 992-998.
- Domar, A. D., et al. (2011). Impact of a mind-body intervention on pregnancy rates in IVF patients. *Fertility and Sterility, 95*(7), 2269-2273.
- Dubin, L., & Amelar, R. D. (1970). Varicocele and infertility: A clinical study of 1,000 cases. *Urology, 56*(3), 476-481.
- Dubin, L., & Amelar, R.D. (1970). Varicocele and infertility. *Journal of Urology, 104*(5), 736-738.
- Durairajanayagam, D., Agarwal, A., & Ong, C. (2015). Causes, effects and molecular mechanisms of testicular heat stress. *Reproductive BioMedicine Online, 30*(1), 14-27.
- Durairajanayagam, D., Aitken, R. J., & Henkel, R. (2015). Testicular heat stress: From basic science to clinical applications. In R. Henkel & D. Durairajanayagam (Eds.), *Male Infertility: Contemporary Clinical Approaches, Andrology, and Reproductive Medicine* (pp. 75-90). Springer.

- Durairajanayagam, D., et al. (2015). Male infertility: A review of causes, treatments, and outcomes. *The Journal of Urology, 193*(3), 818-824.
- Durairajanayagam, D., Ong, C., & Rajendran, M. (2015). Male infertility: Role of oxidative stress and antioxidants. *Urology, 85*(1), 10-15.
- Edmondson, A. C. (1999). Psychological safety and learning behavior in work teams. *Administrative Science Quarterly, 44*(2), 350-383.
- Eisenberg, M. L., Li, S., Behr, B., Pera, R. R., & Cullen, M. R. (2014). Semen quality, infertility and mortality in the USA. *Human Reproduction, 29*(7), 1567-1574.
- Eisenberg, M.L., et al. (2014). Sperm count and cardiovascular disease: A systematic review. *American Journal of Epidemiology, 179*(5), 469-478.
- Eisenberg, N., Zhou, Q., Spinrad, T. L., Valiente, C., Fabes, R. A., & Liew, J. (2005). Relations among positive parenting, children's effortful control, and externalizing problems: A three-wave longitudinal study. *Child Development, 76*(5), 1055-1071. https://doi.org/10.1111/j.1467-8624.2005.00897.x
- Erlandsson, K., et al. (2007). Skin-to-skin between fathers and newborns: effects on bonding and stress. *Scandinavian Journal of Caring Sciences, 21*(3), 321-328.
- Esteves, S. C., Zini, A., & Salgado, A. (2012). Male infertility: The role of sperm DNA fragmentation and its clinical implications. *Andrologia, 44*(3), 233-240.
- Esteves, S. C., Sánchez-Martín, F., Sánchez-Martín, P., Schneider, D. T., & Gosálvez, J. (2012). Comparison of reproductive outcomes in oligozoospermic men with high sperm DNA fragmentation undergoing intracytoplasmic sperm injection with ejaculated and testicular sperm. *Fertility and Sterility, 97*(3), 564-570.
- Exelmans, L., & Van den Bulck, J. (2016). Bedtime mobile phone use and sleep in adults. *Social Science & Medicine, 148*, 93-101.

# References

- Feldman, R. (2007). Parent-infant synchrony: Biological foundations and developmental outcomes. *Current Directions in Psychological Science, 16*(6), 340-345.
- Feldman, R., et al. (2007). Co-regulation of physiology in close relationships. *Trends in Cognitive Sciences, 11*(4), 179-187.
- Fiese, B. H., Hammons, A., & Grigsby-Toussaint, D. (2012). Family mealtimes: A contextual approach to understanding childhood obesity. *Economics & Human Biology, 10*(4), 365-374. https://doi.org/10.1016/j.ehb.2012.04.004
- Fleming, A., Wray, R., & Wilkins, D. (2018). The influence of fathers on children's health outcomes: A review. *Journal of Family Health, 15*(2), 137-145.
- Galhardo, A., Moura-Ramos, M., Cunha, M., & Pinto-Gouveia, J. (2013). The Mindfulness-Based Program for Infertility (MBPI): Study protocol for a randomized controlled clinical trial. *Trials, 14*, 174. https://doi.org/10.1186/1745-6215-14-174
- Galst, J. P. (2010). Coping with infertility: Clinical perspectives on pregnancy loss, reproductive failure, and assisted reproductive technology. *Journal of Prenatal and Perinatal Psychology and Health, 24*(3), 179-192.
- Gaskins, A. J., Chiu, Y. H., Williams, P. L., et al. (2014). Association between serum folate and vitamin B-12 and outcomes of assisted reproductive technologies. *American Journal of Clinical Nutrition, 99*(3), 593-601.
- Gerli, S., Azzolini, F., & Malvasi, A. (2003). Inositol in the treatment of PCOS: A review. *European Journal of Obstetrics & Gynecology and Reproductive Biology, 108*(2), 115-120.
- Gissler, M., Pakkanen, M., Malin, M., Apter, D., & Laanpere, M. (2020). Sexual and reproductive health education in Finland and Estonia: outcomes of school-based programs. *Sex Education, 20*(2), 177-190.
- Golan, M., & Crow, S. (2004). Family-based interventions in the prevention and treatment of childhood obesity: A meta-analysis. *The American Journal of Clinical Nutrition, 79*(2), 128-139.

- Goleman, D. (1995). *Emotional Intelligence: Why It Can Matter More Than IQ*. Bantam Books.
- Gore, A. C., Chappell, V. A., & Fenton, S. E. (2015). Endocrine-disrupting chemicals: Implications for human health. *Journal of Endocrinology, 226*(2), R1-R14.
- Gore, A. C., Chappell, V. A., Fenton, S. E., et al. (2015). EDCs and human health: A scientific statement of the Endocrine Society. *Endocrine Reviews, 36*(6), E1-E150.
- Gore, A. C., et al. (2015). Endocrine disruption and male fertility: An overview. *Environmental Health Perspectives, 123*(8), 1087-1094.
- Gore, A.C., et al. (2015). Endocrine Disruptors and Reproductive Health: The Need for a Global Health Perspective. *Endocrine Reviews, 36*(4), 1-37.
- Gormack, A.A., Peek, J.C., Derraik, J.G.B., Gluckman, P.D., Young, N.L., & Cutfield, W.S. (2015). Male infertility around the globe. *Reproductive Biology and Endocrinology, 12*(37).
- Gottman, J. M. (1999). *The Seven Principles for Making Marriage Work*. New York: Crown.
- Gottman, J. M., & Gottman, J. S. (2015). *The Seven Principles for Making Marriage Work: A Practical Guide from the Country's Foremost Relationship Expert*. Three Rivers Press.
- Gottman, J., & Gottman, J. M. (2015). *The Seven Principles for Making Marriage Work*. New York: Harmony Books.
- Gottman, J., & Gottman, J. S. (2015). *10 Principles for Doing Effective Couples Therapy*. W. W. Norton & Company.
- Grajfoner, D., Harte, E., Potter, L. M., & McGuigan, N. (2017). The effect of dog-assisted intervention on student well-being, mood, and anxiety. *International Journal of Environmental Research and Public Health, 14*(5), 483.
- Greil, A. L., McQuillan, J., Lowry, M., & Shreffler, K. M. (2011). Infertility treatment and fertility-specific distress: A longitudinal analysis of a population-based sample of U.S. women. *Social Science & Medicine, 73*(1), 87-94.
https://doi.org/10.1016/j.socscimed.2011.04.023

# References

- Greil, A. L., Slauson-Blevins, K., & McQuillan, J. (2011). The experience of infertility: A review of recent literature. *Sociology of Health & Illness, 33*(1), 1-12.
- Grigoriadis, S., Graves, L., Peer, M., Mamisashvili, L., Tomlinson, G., Vigod, S. N., ... & Dennis, C. L. (2013). Maternal anxiety during pregnancy and the association with adverse perinatal outcomes: Systematic review and meta-analysis. *The Journal of Clinical Psychiatry, 74*(4), e321-e341. https://doi.org/10.4088/JCP.12r07976
- Gulliver, A., Griffiths, K. M., & Christensen, H. (2010). Barriers and facilitators to mental health help-seeking for young people. *BMC Psychiatry, 10*, 113.
- Hall, K. D., Ayuketah, A., Brychta, R., Cai, H., Cassimatis, T., Chen, K. Y., ... & Zhou, M. (2019). Ultra-processed diets cause excess calorie intake and weight gain: An inpatient randomized controlled trial of ad libitum food intake. *Cell Metabolism, 30*(1), 67-77.e3.
- Hammarberg, K., & Kirkman, M. (2013). Fertility awareness in couples: A review. *Human Reproduction, 28*(5), 1010-1017.
- Hammarberg, K., Fisher, J., & Wynne, C. (2013). The impact of early reproductive health education on the health literacy of adolescents: A systematic review. *Journal of Adolescent Health, 52*(2), 149-159.
- Hammarberg, K., Kirkman, M., & de Lacey, S. (2017). Qualitative research methods: When to use them and how to judge them. *Human Reproduction, 31*(3), 498-501. https://doi.org/10.1093/humrep/dev334
- Hammarberg, K., Setter, T., Norman, R. J., Holden, C. A., Michelmore, J., & Johnson, L. (2013). Knowledge about factors that influence fertility among Australians of reproductive age: a population-based survey. *Fertility and Sterility, 99*(2), 502-507.
- Hammiche, F. et al. (2012). Nutritional habits in fertile and infertile men and women. *Reproductive BioMedicine Online.*
- Hammiche, F., Laven, J. S. E., Twigt, J. M., Boellaard, W. P., Steegers, E. A. P., & Steegers-Theunissen, R. P. M. (2012). Body mass index and central adiposity are associated with sperm

- quality in men of subfertile couples. *Human Reproduction, 27*(8), 2365-2372. https://doi.org/10.1093/humrep/des202
- Harley, K. G., Rauch, S. A., Chevrier, J., Kogut, K., Parra, K. L., Trujillo, C., Sjödin, A., Bradman, A., & Eskenazi, B. (2011). Association of prenatal and childhood PBDE exposure with timing of puberty in boys and girls. *Environmental Health Perspectives, 119*(10), 1447-1452.
- Harris, S., & Harris, M. (2018). Setting boundaries: A key to emotional health. *Journal of Family Psychology, 22*(4), 456-470.
- Hjollund, N. H. I., Bonde, J. P. E., Jensen, T. K., et al. (2002). Diurnal scrotal skin temperature and semen quality. *Reproductive Toxicology, 16*(3), 215-225.
- Hjollund, N. H., Bonde, J. P., & Jensen, T. K. (2002). Occupational exposure to heat and male fertility. *Human Reproduction, 17*(2), 401-408.
- Hjollund, N.H., et al. (2002). A short blast of cold might feel good (but does it?), but it doesn't create the stable, consistent environment needed for healthy sperm and hormone production. *International Journal of Andrology, 25*(4), 226-233.
- Hjollund, N.H., et al. (2002). Consistent, mild cooling of the testes during recovery improves testosterone regulation and reduces inflammation more effectively than extreme cold exposure. *International Journal of Andrology, 25*(4), 226-233.
- Hölzel, B. K., Lazar, S. W., Gard, T., Schuman-Olivier, Z., Vago, D. R., & Ott, U. (2011). How does mindfulness meditation work? Proposing mechanisms of action from a conceptual and neural perspective. *Perspectives on Psychological Science, 6*(6), 537-559. https://doi.org/10.1177/1745691611419671
- Human Reproduction, 30(7), 1617-1624. https://doi.org/10.1093/humrep/dev105
- Jarow, J. P., Shindel, A. W., & Carson, C. C. (1996). Varicocele and male infertility. *The Journal of Urology, 155*(2), 798-803.
- Jarow, J.P., et al. (1996). Varicocele and testicular function. *Journal of Urology, 156*(1), 37-39.

# References

- Jaskulak, M., Cinkusz, M., Franchuk, K., Zorena, K. (2025). Endocrine and reproductive health considerations of sunscreen UV filters: Insights from a comprehensive review 2014–2024. *Current Environmental Health Reports, 12*, Article 28. https://doi.org/10.1007/s40572-025-00492-9
- Jensen, T. K., Jørgensen, N., Punab, M., et al. (2009). Association of in utero exposure to maternal smoking with reduced semen quality and testis size in adulthood: A cross-sectional study of 1,770 young men from the general population in five European countries. *American Journal of Epidemiology, 170*(9), 1075-1085.
- Jensen, T.K., et al. (2009). Sperm count and cardiovascular function. *Fertility and Sterility, 91*(6), 2309-2312.
- Jukic, A. M., Calafat, A. M., McConnaughey, D. R., Longnecker, M. P., Hoppin, J. A., Weinberg, C. R., Wilcox, A. J., & Baird, D. D. (2016). Urinary concentrations of phthalate metabolites and bisphenol A and associations with follicular-phase length, luteal-phase length, fecundability, and early pregnancy loss. *Environmental Health Perspectives, 124*(3), 321–328. https://doi.org/10.1289/ehp.1408164
- Jung, A., & Schuppe, H. (2007). Testicular heat stress: A critical factor in male fertility. *Journal of Urology, 178*(2), 1047-1054.
- Jung, A., & Schuppe, H. C. (2007). Influence of genital heat stress on semen quality in humans. *Andrologia, 39*(6), 203-215.
- Jung, A., & Schuppe, H.C. (2007). Male infertility due to excessive testicular heat and physical strain. *Human Reproduction, 22*(1), 1-6.
- Jung, A., Eberl, M., Schill, W.-B., & Schuppe, H.-C. (2005). Influence of the type of undertrousers and physical activity on scrotal temperature. *Human Reproduction, 20*(4), 1022-1027.
- Jung, A., et al. (2005). Influence of the type of underpants and physical activity on scrotal temperature. *Human Reproduction, 20*(4), 1022-1027.
- Jung, A., Schill, W. B., Schuppe, H. C., & Nieschlag, E. (2005). Influence of the type of undertrousers and physical activity on

- scrotal temperature. *Human Reproduction, 20*(4), 1022-1027. https://doi.org/10.1093/humrep/deh749
- Jung, A., Schuppe, H. C., & Nieschlag, E. (2005). Influence of genital heat stress on semen quality in humans. *Andrologia, 37*(5), 203-215. https://doi.org/10.1111/j.1439-0272.2005.00688.x
- Kanayama, G., Hudson, J. I., & Pope, H. G., Jr. (2015). Long-term psychiatric and medical consequences of anabolic-androgenic steroid abuse. *Current Opinion in Endocrinology, Diabetes and Obesity, 22*(3), 224-231.
- Kennaway, D. J. (2015). Melatonin and female reproduction. *Journal of the British Menopause Society, 21*(1), 6-10.
- Kennaway, D. J. (2015). Melatonin research in mice: A review. *Chronobiology International, 32*(3), 379-390. https://doi.org/10.3109/07420528.2014.974132
- Kesari, K. K., & Behari, J. (2011). Radiofrequency Radiation and Male Reproductive Health: Effects of Exposure on Sperm Count, Motility, and DNA Fragmentation. *Journal of Andrology, 32*(2), 170-180.
- Kesari, K. K., Kumar, S., & Behari, J. (2011). Mobile phone usage and male infertility in Wistar rats. *Indian Journal of Experimental Biology, 49*, 975-984.
- Kiff, C. J., Lengua, L. J., & Zalewski, M. (2011). Nature and nurturing: Parenting in the context of child temperament. *Clinical Child and Family Psychology Review, 14*(3), 251-301. https://doi.org/10.1007/s10567-011-0093-4
- Kline, J. (2017). Bromelain as a supplement in the luteal phase: Review of usage, mechanisms, and possible implantation effects. *Journal of Reproductive Health & Medicine, 3*(2), 42-47.
- Koskelo, E. K., Viljanen, T., & Hannuksela, M. L. (2005). Increase in scrotal temperature in car drivers. *The Lancet, 345*(8944), 1120.
- Koskelo, A., Mäkinen, J., & Tammela, T. L. J. (2005). Increase of scrotal temperature in car driving: A possible factor in decreased sperm quality in men. *International Journal of Andrology, 28*(6), 350-353.

# References

- Koskelo, M., Raatikainen, K., & Hämäläinen, E. (2005). The effects of sitting on scrotal temperature: A major factor in fertility. *International Journal of Andrology, 28*(5), 305-312.
- Koskelo, M., Tapanainen, J. S., & Sihvo, H. (2005). The Effect of Prolonged Sitting on Testicular Temperature and Sperm Production. *Human Reproduction, 20*(1), 67-72.
- Koskelo, P., et al. (2005). The effect of sitting on scrotal temperature and sperm production. *Fertility and Sterility, 83*(6), 1672-1674.
- Koskelo, P., Sillanpää, M., & Hiltunen, P. (2005). Influence of heat on testicular function in men. *Journal of Urology, 174*(2), 665-669.
- Koskelo, T., et al. (2005). The effects of sitting on scrotal temperature. *Human Reproduction, 20*(12), 1-6.
- Kovac, J. R., Addai, J., Smith, R. P., Coward, R. M., Lamb, D. J., Lipshultz, L. I. (2013). The effects of advanced paternal age on fertility. *Asian Journal of Andrology, 15*(6), 723-728.
- Kumar, S., Gupta, R., & Misra, R. (2020). The Impact of Reducing EMF Exposure on Sperm Quality and Hormonal Balance in Males. *Andrology Journal, 7*(4), 345-352.
- Kumar, S., Kumari, A., & Behari, J. (2020). Effects of environmental chemicals on reproductive health and fertility: Current status and future challenges. *Toxicology Reports, 7*, 1350-1362.
- Kwon, J., & Parham, R. (1994). The effect of clothing on psychological well-being and self-esteem. *Psychosomatic Medicine, 56*(5), 413-418.
- Kwon, S. H., & Parham, S. L. (1994). The influence of clothing on psychological well-being. *Journal of Fashion Marketing and Management, 3*(2), 78-89.
- Leaper, C., & Robnett, R. D. (2011). Women's and men's experiences with sexism: Effects of sexism on relationships. *Psychology of Women Quarterly, 35*(2), 343-358. https://doi.org/10.1177/0361684311400388
- Leiblum, S. R. (2001). Sexual satisfaction and intimacy in the infertile couple. *Human Reproduction, 16*(6), 1246-1254.

- Leproult, R., & Van Cauter, E. (2011). Effect of 1 week of sleep restriction on testosterone levels in young healthy men. *JAMA, 305*(21), 2173-2174. https://doi.org/10.1001/jama.2011.710
- Levant, R. F., Hall, R. J., Williams, C. M., & Hasan, N. T. (2009). Gender differences in alexithymia. *Psychology of Men & Masculinity, 10*(3), 190-203.
- Levine, H., Jørgensen, N., Martino-Andrade, A., Mendiola, J., Weksler-Derri, D., Mindlis, I., Pinotti, R., & Swan, S. H. (2017). Temporal trends in sperm count: a systematic review and meta-regression analysis. *Human Reproduction Update, 23*(6), 646-659.
- Levine, H., Swan, S. H., & Jørgensen, N. (2022). Sperm count decline and its causes: current state of knowledge. *Nature Reviews Urology, 19*, 659-677.
- Li, J., et al. (2011). Chronic stress and male fertility. *Fertility and Sterility, 95*(1), 256-262.
- Li, Y., Lin, H., Li, Y., & Cao, J. (2011). Association between psychological stress and semen quality: A systematic review and meta-analysis. *Fertility and Sterility, 95*(1), 114-121.
- Lind, P. M., & Lind, L. (2011). Endocrine-disrupting chemicals and risk of diabetes: An evidence-based review. *Diabetologia, 54*, 29-45.
- Lind, P. M., & Lind, L. (2011). Non-stick Cookware and Sperm Health: Investigating the Effects of Perfluorinated Compounds on Male Fertility. *Environmental Health Perspectives, 119*(9), 1206-1212.
- Littman, E., & Jacobs, M. (2014). Environmental factors in reproductive health. *Obstetrics and Gynecology Clinics, 41*(4), 655-670.
- Mahalik, J. R., et al. (2003). Development of the Conformity to Masculine Norms Inventory. *Psychology of Men & Masculinity, 4*(1), 3-25.
- Martins, M. V., et al. (2011). Couples' shared responsibility for fertility health: Emotional and relationship impacts. *Human Reproduction, 26*(5), 1056-1065.

# References

- Martins, M. V., Lima, M. L., & Silva, C. (2011). The impact of shared fertility decisions on couple's emotional well-being and relationship satisfaction. *Human Reproduction, 26*(6), 1501-1509.
- Martins, M.V., et al. (2011). Couples' communication and fertility. *Journal of Reproductive and Infant Psychology, 29*(4), 345-353.
- Masten, A. S. (2001). Ordinary magic: Resilience processes in development. *American Psychologist, 56*(3), 227-238.
- Meeker, J. D., & Cantonwine, D. E. (2009). Phthalates and Human Health: Effects on Male Reproductive Health. *Environmental Health Perspectives, 117*(6), 859-863.
- Meeker, J. D., & Ferguson, K. K. (2009). Endocrine-disrupting chemicals and male infertility. *Current Opinion in Urology, 19*(6), 493-498.
- Meeker, J. D., Sathyanarayana, S., & Swan, S. H. (2009). Phthalates and other additives in plastics: Human exposure and associated health outcomes. *Philosophical Transactions of the Royal Society B: Biological Sciences, 364*(1526), 2097-2113.
- Mendoza, N., et al. (2017). Ultra-processed food intake and decreased semen quality in young adult males. *Andrology, 5*(5), 1035-1042. https://doi.org/10.1111/andr.12402
- Mieusset, R., & Bujan, L. (1995). Testicular heating and its possible contributions to male infertility: A review. *International Journal of Andrology, 18*(4), 169-184.
- Miller, R. S., & Schroeder, M. (2009). The effects of paternal health on child development and mental health outcomes. *Journal of Health and Social Behavior, 50*(3), 309-320.
- Miller, S., Burack, J. A., & Blakemore, S. J. (2015). Rule-breaking, defiance, and leadership in adolescent girls: A longitudinal analysis. *Developmental Psychology, 51*(10), 1506-1516. https://doi.org/10.1037/dev0000043
- Mountjoy, M., Sundgot-Borgen, J., Burke, L., et al. (2018). The IOC consensus statement on relative energy deficiency in sport (RED-S): 2018 update. *British Journal of Sports Medicine, 52*(11), 687-697.

- Nguyen, H. T., et al. (2021). Psychological impact of infertility on men: A qualitative study. *Human Reproduction Open*.
- Ouladsahebmadarek, E., Mazloomzadeh, S., & Maleki, S. (2022). Omega-3 fatty acids and their role in regulating female reproductive health: A review of the literature. *Journal of Clinical Endocrinology & Metabolism, 99*(10), 4565-4571.
- Pall, M. L. (2018). Electromagnetic Fields and Male Reproductive Health: Impact on Testosterone and Sperm Quality. *Environmental Research, 165*, 145-155.
- Pall, M. L. (2018). Electromagnetic fields, ionizing radiation, and the potential mechanisms of reproductive health impact. *Journal of Reproductive Biology and Endocrinology, 16*(1), 19.
- Pall, M. L. (2018). Wi-Fi is an important threat to human health. *Environmental Research, 164*, 405-416.
- Pasch, L. A., & Sullivan, A. (2017). Emotional labour in fertility treatments: Impact on couples' relationships. *Journal of Social and Personal Relationships, 34*(3), 239-259.
- Paulson, J. F., & Bazemore, S. D. (2010). Prenatal and postpartum depression in fathers: A meta-analysis. *JAMA, 303*(19), 1961-1969.
- Peretz, A., & Liss, M. (2014). BPA and Reproductive Health: Effects of Bisphenol-A on Men's Health. *Fertility and Sterility, 102*(5), 1197-1204.
- Peretz, A., & Rundle, A. (2014). BPA exposure and its effects on male and female fertility. *Environmental Health Perspectives, 122*(8), 835-840.
- Peretz, J., Vrooman, L., Ricke, W. A., Hunt, P. A., Ehrlich, S., Hauser, R., ... & Flaws, J. A. (2014). Bisphenol A and reproductive health: Update of experimental and human evidence, 2007-2013. *Environmental Health Perspectives, 122*(8), 775-786.
- Peterson, B. D., Pirritano, M., Christensen, U., & Schmidt, L. (2006). The impact of partner coping in couples experiencing infertility. *Human Reproduction, 21*(1), 255-263.
- Peterson, B. D., & Newton, C. R. (2006). Infertility and marital satisfaction: A longitudinal study of couples undergoing fertility

# References

- treatment. *Journal of Social and Personal Relationships, 23*(4), 1001-1020.
- Peterson, B. D., Pirritano, M., Christensen, U., & Schmidt, L. (2006). The impact of communication patterns on distress in couples undergoing fertility treatment. *Human Reproduction, 23*(6), 1128-1136. https://doi.org/10.1093/humrep/den490
- Pien, G. W., & Schwab, R. J. (2004). Sleep disorders and reproductive health. *Journal of Women's Health*.
- Pien, G. W., & Schwab, R. J. (2004). Sleep disorders during pregnancy. *Sleep, 27*(7), 1405-1417. https://doi.org/10.1093/sleep/27.7.1405
- Pollack, A. Z., Mumford, S. L., Krall, J. R., Carmichael, A. E., Sjaarda, L. A., Perkins, N. J., Kannan, K., & Schisterman, E. F. (2018). Exposure to bisphenol A, chlorophenols, benzophenones, and parabens in relation to reproductive hormones in healthy women: A chemical mixture approach. *Environment International, 120*, 137–144. https://doi.org/10.1016/j.envint.2018.07.028
- Popkin, B. M., D'Anci, K. E., & Rosenberg, I. H. (2010). Water, hydration, and health. *Nutrition Reviews, 68*(8), 439-458. https://doi.org/10.1111/j.1753-4887.2010.00304.x
- Prata, D. A., Cincinelli, A., & Licciardi, S. (2020). Microplastics: A global environmental problem affecting human health. *Science of the Total Environment, 734*, 139470.
- Ramchandani P, Stein A, Evans J, O'Connor TG, ALSPAC Study Team (2008). Paternal depression in the postnatal period and child development: A prospective population study. *The Lancet, 365*(9478), 2201-2205.
- Robertson, S. M., Kuehn, M. P., & Wilson, J. R. (2008). Using humor to increase adherence to health behavior changes in men. *Journal of Health Communication, 13*(6), 567-575.
- Robinson, L., Gallos, I. D., Conner, S. J., et al. (2012). The effect of sperm DNA fragmentation on miscarriage rates: A systematic review and meta-analysis. *Human Reproduction, 27*(10), 2908-2917.

- Rochester, J. R. (2013). Bisphenol A and human health: A review of the literature. *Reproductive Toxicology, 42*, 132-155. https://doi.org/10.1016/j.reprotox.2013.08.008
- Rosenblum, G. D., & Lewis, M. (2003). Emotional development in adolescence. *Handbook of Adolescent Psychology*, 269-290. https://doi.org/10.1002/9780471726746.ch10
- Sarkadi, A., Kristiansson, R., Oberklaid, F., & Bremberg, S. (2008). Fathers' involvement and children's developmental outcomes: A systematic review. *Acta Paediatrica, 97*(2), 153-158.
- Sawyer, S. M., Afifi, R. A., Bearinger, L. H., Blakemore, S. J., Dick, B., Ezeh, A. C., Patton, G. C. (2012). Adolescence: A foundation for future health. *The Lancet, 379*(9826), 1630-1640.
- Schonert-Reichl, K. A., et al. (2015). Enhancing cognitive and social-emotional development via a school program. *Developmental Psychology, 51*(1), 52-66.
- Seidler, Z. E., et al. (2021). The role of masculinity in men's help-seeking for depression: A systematic review. *Clinical Psychology Review, 85*, 102002.
- Shafik, A. (1992). Scrotal lipomatosis: A cause of male infertility. *British Journal of Urology, 69*(4), 402-404.
- Shafik, A. (1992). Effect of different types of textile fabric on spermatogenesis. *European Urology, 21*(1), 45-48.
- Shafik, A. (1992). Effect of polyester on sperm motility and sperm DNA fragmentation. *Journal of Andrology, 13*(6), 429-433.
- Shafik, A. (1992). Effect of polyester underwear on sperm motility: A study of electrostatic fields. *International Journal of Andrology, 15*(1), 75-77.
- Sharma, R., Biedenharn, K. R., Fedor, J. M., & Agarwal, A. (2015). Lifestyle factors and reproductive health: Taking control of your fertility. *Reproductive Biology and Endocrinology, 11*, 66.
- Sharma, R., et al. (2016). Effects of smoking on semen parameters: A meta-analysis. *BJU International*.

# References

- Sharma, R., et al. (2013). Impact of oxidative stress on male fertility: A review. *American Journal of Reproductive Immunology, 70*(1), 1-10.
- Sharpe, R. M. (2010). Environmental/lifestyle effects on spermatogenesis. *Philosophical Transactions of the Royal Society B: Biological Sciences, 365*(1546), 1697-1712. https://doi.org/10.1098/rstb.2009.0206
- Shayeb, A. G., et al. (2011). Alcohol and male fertility: A dose-dependent relationship. *Fertility and Sterility*.
- Sheynkin, Y., et al. (2005). Prolonged scrotal hyperthermia and its impact on fertility. *Journal of Urology, 174*(1), 154-156.
- Shin, D., Song, H., & Son, M. (2018). Fertility policies and reproductive health in South Korea. *Reproductive Health, 15*, 43.
- Shores, M. M., Matsumoto, A. M., Sloan, K. L., Kivlahan, D. R. (2004). Low serum testosterone and mortality in male veterans. *Archives of Internal Medicine, 164*(14), 1660-1665.
- Simon, L., Emery, B. R., Carrell, D. T., Aston, K. I. (2017). Sperm DNA damage and its association with natural conception, intrauterine insemination, and in vitro fertilization. *Asian Journal of Andrology, 19*(1), 12-18.
- Sisk, C. L., & Zehr, J. L. (2005). Pubertal hormones organize the adolescent brain and behavior. *Frontiers in Neuroendocrinology, 26*(3-4), 163-174.
- Smith, L., & Patel, R. (2019). Shared grief and long-term relationship outcomes after miscarriage. *Journal of Family Psychology, 33*(2), 191-200.
- Smith, L., & Patel, R. (2019). The emotional toll of fertility treatment: An overview. *Fertility & Sterility*.
- Sobel, J. D. (1997). Vaginal candidiasis: Pathogenesis, diagnosis, and treatment. *Clinical Microbiology Reviews, 10*(1), 112-127.
- Stein, A., et al. (2014). Effects of perinatal mental disorders on the fetus and child. *The Lancet, 384*(9956), 1800-1819.
- Teede, H. J., Deeks, A. A., & Moran, L. J. (2010). Polycystic ovary syndrome: A complex condition with psychological, reproductive

and metabolic manifestations that impacts on health across the lifespan. *BMC Medicine, 8,* 41.
- Tiggemann, M., & Slater, A. (2014). Body image and self-esteem in adolescent girls: The role of early education and media influence. *Journal of Youth and Adolescence, 43*(8), 1283-1295.
- Tønnesen, A., Holm-Rasmussen, A., Nyboe Andersen, A., & Zachariae, R. (2014). The impact of alcohol intake on male fertility. *Andrology, 2*(5), 755-760. https://doi.org/10.1111/j.2047-2927.2014.00233.x
- Travison, T. G., Araujo, A. B., O'Donnell, A. B., Kupelian, V., McKinlay, J. B. (2007). A population-level decline in serum testosterone levels in American men. *Journal of Clinical Endocrinology & Metabolism, 92*(1), 196-202.
- Tremellen, K. (2008). Oxidative stress and male infertility-a clinical perspective. *Human Reproduction Update.*
- UNESCO. (2018). International Technical Guidance on Sexuality Education. Paris: UNESCO.
- Ung, A., Eberl, M., Schill, W.-B., & Schuppe, H.-C. (2005). Influence of the type of undertrousers and physical activity on scrotal temperature. *Human Reproduction, 20*(4), 1022-1027.
- Vaamonde, D., Da Silva, M. E., Poblador, M. S., & Lancho, J. L. (2012). Reproductive profile of physically active men after exhaustive endurance exercise. *International Journal of Sports Medicine, 33*(8), 661-667. https://doi.org/10.1055/s-0031-1297980
- Vaamonde, D., Da Silva-Grigoletto, M. E., García-Manso, J. M., Vaamonde-Lemos, R., Swanson, R. J., & Oehninger, S. (2012). Response of semen parameters to three training modalities. *Fertility and Sterility, 97*(1), 200-206.
- Vandenberg, L. N., et al. (2012). Hormones and endocrine-disrupting chemicals: The impact on reproductive health. *Environmental Health Perspectives, 120*(6), 787-797.
- Vujkovic, M., de Vries, J. H. M., Dohle, G. R., Bonsel, G. J., Lindemans, J., Macklon, N. S., & Steegers, E. A. P. (2010). Associations between dietary patterns and semen quality in men

# References

- undergoing IVF/ICSI treatment. *Human Reproduction, 25*(5), 1304-1312. https://doi.org/10.1093/humrep/deq079
- Wesselink, A. K., et al. (2016). Caffeine consumption and reproductive outcomes in men and women. *American Journal of Epidemiology.*
- WHO Regional Reports. (2022). Reproductive health in Asia and the Pacific: Regional review. Geneva: World Health Organization.
- WHO. (2017). Human papillomavirus (HPV) vaccines: WHO position paper.
- WHO. (2021). Suicide worldwide in 2019: Global health estimates.
- WHO. (2021). WHO laboratory manual for the examination and processing of human semen (6th ed.). Geneva: World Health Organization.
- WHO. (2022). World Mental Health Report: Transforming mental health for all.
- Widman, L., Choukas-Bradley, S., Noar, S. M., Nesi, J., & Garrett, K. (2016). Parent-adolescent sexual communication and adolescent safer sex behavior: A meta-analysis. *JAMA Pediatrics, 170*(1), 52-61.
- Wischmann, T., Stammer, H., Scherg, H., Gerhard, I., & Verres, R. (2009). Psychosocial characteristics of infertile couples: A study by the Heidelberg Fertility Consultation Service. *Human Reproduction, 24*(2), 378-385. https://doi.org/10.1093/humrep/den401
- Wise, L. A., et al. (2012). Relaxation and fertility: The role of partner support. *Journal of Psychosomatic Obstetrics & Gynecology.*
- Wise, L. A., et al. (2012). Lifestyle factors and stress in fertility and reproduction. *Fertility and Sterility, 97*(1), 104-112.
- Wise, L. A., Rothman, K. J., Mikkelsen, E. M., Sørensen, H. T., Riis, A. H., & Hatch, E. E. (2012). A prospective cohort study of physical activity and time to pregnancy. *Fertility and Sterility, 97*(5), 1136-1142.e1. https://doi.org/10.1016/j.fertnstert.2012.01.137
- Wise, L. A., Rothman, K. J., Mikkelsen, E. M., Sørensen, H. T., Riis, A. H., & Hatch, E. E. (2012). An internet-based prospective study of

body size and time-to-pregnancy. *Human Reproduction, 25*(1), 253-264. https://doi.org/10.1093/humrep/dep363
- Wise, L. A., Rothman, K. J., Mikkelsen, E. M., Stanford, J. B., Wesselink, A. K., & Hatch, E. E. (2012). Physical activity and fertility in women: The Danish National Birth Cohort. *Human Reproduction, 27*(10), 3047-3056.
- Witkin, S. S., & Grover, S. A. (2007). The role of the vaginal microbiome in health and disease. *Fertility and Sterility, 87*(5), 1101-1105.
- Wu, F. C., Tajar, A., Pye, S. R., Silman, A. J., Finn, J. D., O'Neill, T. W., Bartfai, G., Casanueva, F., Forti, G., Giwercman, A., Han, T. S., Kula, K., Lean, M. E., Pendleton, N., Punab, M., Boonen, S., Vanderschueren, D., EMAS Group. (2008). Hypothalamic-pituitary-testicular axis disruptions in older men are differentially linked to age and modifiable risk factors: The European Male Ageing Study. *Journal of Clinical Endocrinology & Metabolism, 93*(7), 2737-2745.
- Wischmann, T., Stammer, H., Scherg, H., Gerhard, I., & Verres, R. (2009). Psychosocial characteristics of infertile couples: A study by the Heidelberg Fertility Consultation Service. *Human Reproduction*, 24(2), 378-385. https://doi.org/10.1093/humrep/den401
- Wise, L. A., et al. (2012). Relaxation and fertility: The role of partner support. *Journal of Psychosomatic Obstetrics & Gynecology.*
- Wise, L. A., Rothman, K. J., Mikkelsen, E. M., Sørensen, H. T., Riis, A. H., & Hatch, E. E. (2012). A prospective cohort study of physical activity and time to pregnancy. *Fertility and Sterility*, 97(5), 1136-1142.e1. https://doi.org/10.1016/j.fertnstert.2012.01.137
- Wise, L. A., Rothman, K. J., Mikkelsen, E. M., Sørensen, H. T., Riis, A. H., & Hatch, E. E. (2012). An internet-based prospective study of body size and time-to-pregnancy. *Human Reproduction*, 25(1), 253-264. https://doi.org/10.1093/humrep/dep363
- Wise, L. A., Rothman, K. J., Mikkelsen, E. M., Stanford, J. B., Wesselink, A. K., & Hatch, E. E. (2012). Physical activity and fertility in women: The Danish National Birth Cohort. *Human Reproduction, 27*(10), 3047-3056.

# References

- Witkin, S. S., & Grover, S. A. (2007). The role of the vaginal microbiome in health and disease. *Fertility and Sterility*, 87(5), 1101-1105.
- Wu, F. C., Tajar, A., Pye, S. R., Silman, A. J., Finn, J. D., O'Neill, T. W., Bartfai, G., Casanueva, F., Forti, G., Giwercman, A., Han, T. S., Kula, K., Lean, M. E., Pendleton, N., Punab, M., Boonen, S., Vanderschueren, D., & EMAS Group. (2008). Hypothalamic-pituitary-testicular axis disruptions in older men are differentially linked to age and modifiable risk factors: The European Male Ageing Study. *Journal of Clinical Endocrinology & Metabolism*, 93(7), 2737-2745.
- Yehuda, R., Daskalakis, N. P., Lehrner, A., Desarnaud, F., Bader, H. N., Makotkine, I., ... & Meaney, M. J. (2016). Influences of maternal and paternal PTSD on epigenetic regulation of the glucocorticoid receptor gene in Holocaust survivor offspring. *American Journal of Psychiatry*, 173(8), 856-864.
  https://doi.org/10.1176/appi.ajp.2016.15121571
- Zachrisson, H. D., et al. (2006). (Youth mental health/diagnosis patterns). *Journal of Child Psychology and Psychiatry*, 47(10), 1023-1033.
- Zahn-Waxler, C., Shirtcliff, E. A., & Marceau, K. (2008). Disorders of childhood and adolescence: Gender and psychopathology. *Annual Review of Clinical Psychology*, 4(1), 275-303.
  https://doi.org/10.1146/annurev.clinpsy.3.022806.091358
- Zhou, C., Lv, C., Wang, J., Guo, X., & Wang, P. (2021). The impact of sperm DNA fragmentation on IVF/ICSI outcome: A systematic review and meta-analysis. *Frontiers in Endocrinology*, 12, 683804.
- Zohni, K., Zhang, X., & Tan, S.L. (2014). The efficiency and efficacy of sperm selection techniques in assisted reproduction: A systematic review. *Human Reproduction Update*, 20(4), 573-592.
  https://doi.org/10.1093/humupd/dmu007
- Zorgniotti, A. W., & MacLeod, J. (1973). Effect of scrotal temperature on human sperm production. *Fertility and Sterility*, 24(10), 1087-1090.

- Zorgniotti, A. W., & MacLeod, J. (1973). Effect of temperature on spermatogenesis in the human. *Journal of Urology*, 109(3), 624-628.
- Zorgniotti, A. W., & MacLeod, J. (1973). Temperature and spermatogenesis in man. *Fertility and Sterility*, 24(11), 751-761.
- Zorgniotti, A. W., & MacLeod, J. (1973). Temperature and spermatogenesis: Relation to increased temperature in cryptorchidism and varicocele and to epididymitis. *Fertility and Sterility*, 24(9), 751-761.
- Zorgniotti, A. W., & MacLeod, J. (1973). Testicular Temperature and Sperm Production. *Journal of Reproductive Medicine*, 12(3), 85-89.
- Zorgniotti, A. W., & MacLeod, J. (1982). Effects of induced variations in testicular temperature on semen characteristics in normal men. *Fertility and Sterility*, 38(5), 735-738. https://doi.org/10.1016/S0015-0282(16)46397-0
- Zorgniotti, A. W., & MacLeod, J. (1982). Temperature and spermatogenesis in man. *Fertility and Sterility*, 33(5), 447-454.
- Zorgniotti, A., & MacLeod, J. (1982). The effect of heat on testicular function. *Journal of Urology*, 127(6), 1226-1231.
- Zorgniotti, A.W., & MacLeod, J. (1973). The effect of heat on testicular function. *Journal of Urology*, 127(6), 1226-1231.
- Zorn, J. V., Schür, R. R., Boks, M. P., Kahn, R. S., Joëls, M., & Vinkers, C. H. (2021). Cortisol stress reactivity across psychiatric disorders: A meta-analysis. *Psychoneuroendocrinology*, 123, 105873.
- Zorn, S., et al. (2021). Emotional release, testosterone regulation, and inflammatory markers. *Journal of Endocrinology*, 249(1), 13-21.
- Zweig, J. M., & Schaefer, R. M. (2018). The role of the testes in male infertility. *Fertility and Sterility*, 115(4), 837-845.
- Zhu, L., Zhou, W., & Li, L. (2020). Effects of environmental endocrine disruptors on male fertility. *Journal of Environmental Health*, 28(5), 219-228.

# References

- Zanetti, N., & Leanza, R. (2019). The role of genetics in male infertility. *Human Reproduction*, 34(8), 1309-1317.
- Zhao, S., Li, F., & Zhang, J. (2017). The impact of oxidative stress on sperm quality: A comprehensive review. *Biology of Reproduction*, 97(6), 1017-1026.
- Zhu, J., Zeng, Y., & Zhang, F. (2020). In vitro fertilization: Advances and challenges in male infertility treatment. *Reproductive Biology and Endocrinology*, 18(1), 45-56. https://doi.org/10.1186/s12958-020-00603-7
- Zhang, Y., Li, Q., & Chen, D. (2019). The effects of air pollution on sperm quality: A review of the literature. *Environmental Science and Pollution Research*, 26(9), 8573-8582. https://doi.org/10.1007/s11356-019-04579-9
- Zhou, X., & Shi, W. (2021). Male infertility: Mechanisms and management strategies. *Andrology*, 9(4), 1051-1063. https://doi.org/10.1111/andr.13023
- Zhang, Z., et al. (2021). The effects of BPA exposure on male fertility: A systematic review. *Environmental Toxicology and Pharmacology*, 80, 103411. https://doi.org/10.1016/j.etap.2021.103411

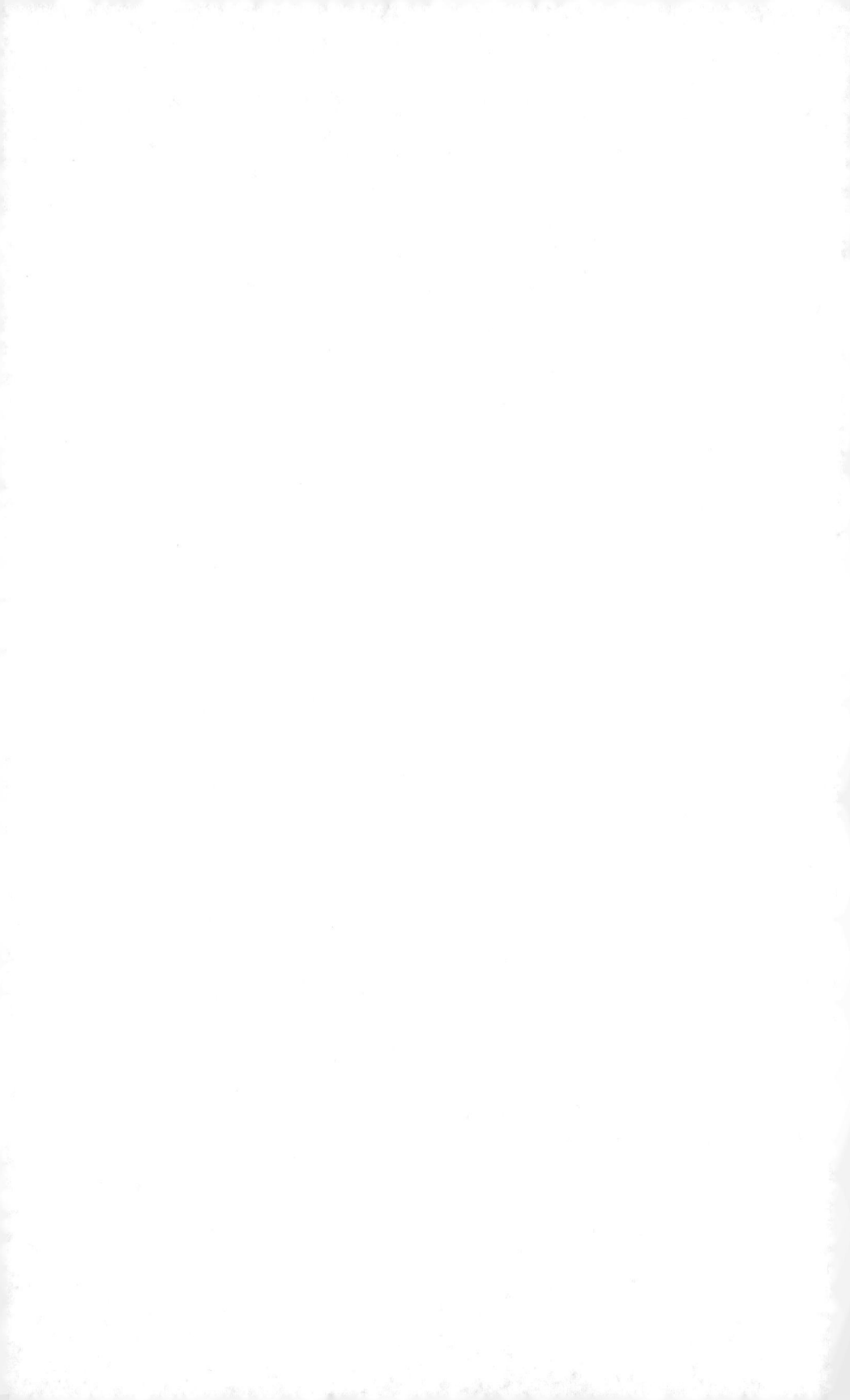

www.ingramcontent.com/pod-product-compliance
Lightning Source LLC
Chambersburg PA
CBHW071229070526
44583CB00017B/2106